Vital & Alive

at 75

A WISE WOMAN'S GUIDE TO LIVING A JOYFUL & HEALTHY LIFE

MAMA RAE

Disclaimer

All the information, techniques, skills and concepts contained within this publication are of the nature of general comment only and are not in any way recommended as individual advice. The intent is to offer a variety of information to provide a wider range of choices now and in the future, recognising that we all have widely diverse circumstances and viewpoints. Should any reader choose to make use of the information herein, this is their decision, and the author and publisher/s do not assume any responsibilities whatsoever under any conditions or circumstances. The author does not take responsibility for the business, financial, personal or other success, results or fulfilment upon the readers' decision to use this information. It is recommended that the reader obtain their own independent advice.

Dedicated to my dear mother and father who both passed away from cancer. It was this that led me on a journey of learning so that I would be able live to a ripe old age, full of spirit and free of illness.

It is also a dedication to my dear friend Cael, who left this Earth at 30 years old and who inspired me to make the most of the years I have left.

Foreword

My mum is one of the most extraordinary people I've ever met.

Am I biased? Perhaps! But just ask the hundreds or thousands of people who have been blessed to meet her and they will tell you that her love radiates out of her like the sun, that they feel warm and relaxed in her presence, that her food is DELICIOUS, and that her sheer presence lights them up. In fact, some would say that her hugs alone are worth travelling the distances of the Earth for (and I agree).

That's who Mama Rae is — and you're about to experience a valuable and long-awaited opportunity to learn from this wise, wacky, and truly wonderful woman about what it takes to LIVE fully with a joyous heart and vital body.

This book is packed full of the greatest wisdom that has changed Mama Rae's life and enabled her to be truly ALIVE in the later years of her Earth journey.

She shares 75 life-changing tips on health, valuable information she believes all human beings deserve to know, and inspiration for living the most meaningful life possible. When applied, Mama Rae's heartfelt messages can turn your life around, lift your spirits, and change your health from the inside out.

I am both proud and overwhelmed with love that my incredibly wise mother has taken the time to write what is, in many senses, her life story so that others may benefit from her magic – and I can't wait for you to read this beautiful book.

Mum: I love your cheeky smile, your wild white hair (that you've so graciously passed down to me through your DNA!), your sense of adventure, your curiosity, and your endless devotion to not only your wellness, but the wellness of the people around you.

To say that you are a blessing to me, and this world is truly, truly an understatement. I love you with my whole heart and I can't wait to see you thrive in the golden years of your life.

With inspiration and deep undying love for my mama,

Emily Gowor
Inspirational Writer, Author & Speaker
(and Mama Rae's youngest chicken)

Table of contents

"You can't go back and change the beginning, but you can start where you are and change the ending."

C S Lewis

Introduction

*I*t is often at the end of one's life when people reflect, that they realise they haven't lived the life of their choosing – it was either chosen for them or it was what they thought they should do. Many people don't live the life of their dreams or even know if it is possible. They realise what was truly important, that they didn't do what they loved, and that they either didn't spend enough time with the people they loved or tell them they loved them.

When my dad was 53, he passed away from cancer, leaving my mum, aged 45 with five children to raise and a herd of dairy cows to milk, morning and night. As a 10-year-old, it was the most devastating thing that could have happened in my life. My dad was my hero, my teacher, and the parent who showed his love for me in the way I understood.

Many people die because of illness rather than old age. Many of the fatal diseases can be linked with and attributed to lifestyle choices which, in reality, could have been avoided. Choices like smoking, alcohol, eating unhealthy food, inactivity, stress, and being overweight often result in conditions like type 2 diabetes, chronic liver disease, irritable bowel syndrome, colitis, heart disease, chronic kidney disease, arthritis, hypertension, and osteoporosis. Of course, there are many more, but I will stop there.

Maybe you are experiencing illness, a lack of wellness or a disease right now, and you're feeling stressed, worried, fearful, or down about it. Perhaps you don't know what to do to heal. However, I believe you don't have to feel despondent or depressed: you can turn your health and your life around. You can do this by making new, educated choices for your body, mind, emotions, and life. Many of the lessons and wisdoms I share in this book will help you to do that. It is my heartfelt intention to share with you the things that have worked for me in maintaining wellness and a zest for life into the golden years of my life – and this is why I have written this book for you.

I was blessed to grow up on a farm where we had enough home-grown meat, vegetables, and orchards close by for me to know what it was like to eat fresh food, to know the delicious taste of a tomato picked straight from the bush or the crunchiness of a juicy apple fresh from the tree. There is nothing like it. The beautiful thing is that the flavour doesn't diminish in your memory. It stays with you.

Once I left home and started shopping for my food in the supermarket, I quickly realised that none of the food I was buying ever tasted like what I was used to at home. I was eager to start growing my own fruit and vegetables as soon as I had the space! Sadly, the reality is that many fruit and vegetables we buy today are far from fresh (even though they are sold to us as being "fresh"). They are kept in cold storage for months before they even reach the supermarket shelves. It is certainly an understatement to say that they taste as fresh as the real thing.

I know many people believe that living a healthy lifestyle is expensive, time-consuming, and hard work to keep up. But the truth is, it is easy when you know how! It isn't about being perfect, it's about changing one small habit at a time and remembering that every decision you make for your wellness is an act of self-care and self-love. We create wellness not with one big action but rather through a series of many small decisions and actions: thousands of them, in fact.

For those of you who want to make changes toward a healthier lifestyle, this book will help you to do that. Choose one change or new habit that resonates with you and try it out for a couple of weeks. Make changes to suit yourself and make a note of any differences or developments you see or feel in yourself. Most importantly, acknowledge yourself for making the effort to improve your life by improving your state of health!

In this book, you will not only find knowledge and wisdom about eating, food, and nutrition. I also explore attitudes and ways of thinking that, if you choose to follow, will allow you to live a healthier and more rewarding life. I don't want anyone to fall to an illness that could have been avoided. To me, that seems a waste of a productive, purposeful, meaningful, and interesting life.

I decided sometime after my dad's passing that I would do all I could to learn what I needed to live a healthy life, free of disease, and with an exuberant enjoyment of my time on this planet. To date, I have been able to do that. I haven't been ill, and I haven't needed to see a doctor since 1986. I don't wear glasses, and I will continue to do all the things I am doing to ensure that I live the rest of my years with boundless energy, enthusiasm, and joy.

My dear friend, that is what I desperately want for you. It may help you to use a journal to write down your thoughts and track your progress. Then, as you read this book, feel into what resonates with you and try it out – not just once but over several days, a week or perhaps two weeks – and see how you feel. Then try another, and another. Find your unique combination of the health habits that help you to create lasting radiance and joy in your body and life. If I can do it, then I know that you can as well.

My love goes with you on your journey.

Here's to your wellness and radiant health!

With love,

Mama Rae

"Never regret yesterday. Life is in you today, and you make your tomorrow."

L Ron Hubbard

1
Live without regrets

We make choices about our lives every day, from what to eat for lunch to what to do with our career or "What will people think if I do that?" Some choices are easy and require a simple "Yes" or "No". Some need to be thought over in depth, and others? Well, the answers come from your heart, so you know they are the right choices for your future.

The unfortunate truth is that so many people go through their life making choices that end up in regret. They miss that chance to do what they love, give up on the opportunity to fulfil their goals, push their dream to the side, or delay their dreams. Let's make a choice now to change that so that you are one of the people who lives every moment and day with a full heart and spirit.

End-of-life carers have found that people close to the end of their time in this life do not reflect on their business successes or the cars they had or the things they bought, but rather on who they were, what they didn't do, and the impact they had. Their thoughts were more about how they lived their life, not their financial wealth or material possessions.

The most common regrets are:

I wish I had taken better care of myself.

I wish I had given more time to the people I cared most about.

I wish I had not worried so much.

I wish I had not worked so much.

I wish I had been more forgiving.

I wish I had stood up for myself more.

I wish I had stayed in touch with my friends.

I wish I had been more honest.

I wish I had been more fulfilled.

I wish I had lived my life the way I wanted to.

I wish I had lived up to my full potential.

I wish I had not cared so much what other people thought.

I wish I had faced my fears.

I wish I had stopped chasing the wrong things.

I wish I had lived more in the moment.

If your life continues the way it is now, will you be able to say honestly at the end of your life that you have lived your life well? Or are there things you would like to change? Is there something else you would add to the list above? Write a list of things you want to change in your life and then prioritise them. Challenge yourself to take on one a month, remembering that it takes three weeks to establish a new habit. Take action on what truly matters to you.

Make the decision to live fully so that when you do reach the end of your life, you don't regret the choices you made — because you know in your heart and soul that you lived WELL.

When you look at your life in this moment, how are you doing your life?

Do you come home from work wishing it was the weekend already?

What regrets do you have?

What could you do differently?

"The more you are grateful for what you have, the more you will have to be grateful for."

Zig Ziglar

2
Be grateful for what you have

One truly cannot put a monetary value on gratitude: it is an expression of appreciation for what we have in our life, whether that is the people we have around us, where we live, or the people we serve. It is not something we have to think about. It comes from our heart, so we feel it. It is an affirmation of the richness and warmth we feel for having these things in our life. Gratitude starts with noticing the goodness in your life.

Once you start practising gratitude, the powerful effects not only ripple through your body, but to the people you surround yourself with. Lasting changes happen in our prefrontal cortex because of the gratitude we feel. Physiological changes happen through the parasympathetic nervous system (the rest and digest) by slowing the heart rate, stimulating digestion, and calming the body.

Research published in the recent decade has shown that grateful people have fewer common health complaints, such as headaches, digestion issues, respiratory infections, runny noses, dizziness, and sleep problems. Other studies show that people who are grateful experience less stress, feel less pain, and achieve more professionally, as well as having stronger immune systems.

It has been found that people who are grateful are able to communicate better with loved ones when showing their gratitude to one another. Gratitude allows them to voice their feelings more easily when there is a disagreement. Feeling and displaying gratitude makes us want to be better people.

Be grateful for everything that has happened for you in your life, both the negative and positive. The negatives are a lesson for you to learn from; the positives are a blessing – and both give you an opportunity to grow.

Gratitude offers us a way of embracing all that makes our lives what they are. More than just a happy feeling for the parts of our lives currently going well, gratitude allows us to be willing to expand our awareness so that we perceive more of the goodness we are always receiving.

A way to start practising gratitude is to keep a gratitude journal and make notes on anything that brought you joy during the day. This could be expressing gratitude for the people who contributed to your life in some way or the things you noticed happening around you that put a smile on your face. Doing this reminds you of the positive things in your life and can help you to move through any adversity more easily.

What or who are you grateful for today?

Who helped you today?

What happened that made your life a little easier?

Was it simply that you had a moment standing in the sunshine, appreciating its warmth?

"Those who think they have no time for healthy eating, will sooner or later have to find time for illness."

Edward Stanley

3

Embrace healthy eating

I believe that what you eat is one of the most important keys to living a vital, healthy, and joyful life. The right food gives you the energy to get things done; you heal quicker; you strengthen your bones, and you keep your skin, teeth, and eyes healthy, in addition to boosting your immune system.

Unfortunately, after going through more than three years of Covid, many people have changed their diet as a result, generally buying more takeaway food than they did before. Although it is far from common knowledge that nutrition is one of the primary aspects of maintaining a healthy life, it can be tough to find the motivation to stay on top of your diet and fitness goals. Eating healthy meals and staying away from junk food can be quite challenging for anyone.

So, let's dive in and see where it takes us. If you want to change your diet (because you want more vitality and energy to do what you love), perhaps the first thing to look at is your eating habits over the past few months, both good and bad. Once you have a clear picture of your habits, prioritise the ones you would like to change. Start with the most important one first: the one you know would make the greatest impact on your health if you changed it overnight.

It may also be helpful to explore any triggers that cause you to eat unhealthy foods, such as emotional eating. Is it stress at work that causes you to want to snack? Is it the inviting plate of cakes or cookies on the table in the tearoom? Do you rush off to work without having breakfast? Is it that you're not taking the time to plan and prepare what you are going to eat the next day?

Once you are aware of your unhealthy food triggers, you can work on them. Some will be easier, like planning your meals and then shopping only for the food you need. This means once you get home from work, you will know what you are going cook. However, other habits might require a little more effort to overcome.

You can always take your own snacks to work so that you aren't tempted by the unhealthy options. If you find yourself eating crisps or potato chips, then don't walk down that aisle in the supermarket! This will lessen the likelihood that you will buy them in the first place! In fact, avoid any aisles that have unhealthy foods in them.

It is interesting to note that 100 years ago 80% of the food in our supermarkets wasn't there – and much of what is there now contains high levels of salt and sugar, neither of which is healthy when consumed in excess. Salty and sugary foods tend to be addictive and so this is often a strategic move by the food companies to keep you buying their product. Unfortunately for us, it works!

Take it one step at a time and notice the difference each change makes. Be kind to yourself. Habits take time to develop. If you find yourself eating something unhealthy, stop and think about why you did it. Was there anything that triggered this unhealthy eating? Don't be hard on yourself and rather look at it as a misstep on the way to building healthier habits.

What are four things you would like to change?

Identify any triggers that lead you to eat unhealthy foods.

Do you need to learn some basic recipes?

Identify the foods you go to if you are stressed.

"Your need for acceptance will make you invisible."

Jim Carrey

4

Love yourself unconditionally

You probably know the saying, "You cannot love someone until you have learned to love yourself." Unfortunately, this isn't always the easiest thing to do. Many people have unresolved pain from their childhood or teenage years where they were criticised or judged for what they said or did. So as adults, there are many beliefs in our subconscious that are telling us we are stupid, careless, clumsy, selfish, or dumb.

We may have had difficult relationships or painful experiences that make it challenging to love ourselves. The truth is though, we are not our actions. We might have done something thoughtless or dumb, but we, in ourselves, are neither thoughtless nor dumb.

The belief I took on when my father passed away was that I wasn't lovable. The 10-year-old in me thought that if I had been lovable, my dad would have lived instead of dying. While at the time I didn't know that was my belief, later in life it was behind many decisions I made, especially in relationships. I used to leave before my partner did. I also put up a wall to protect my heart, which made it difficult to maintain friendships.

The reality is that it is important that we love ourselves. It means having a good understanding of our weaknesses together with our strengths and to be comfortable with them. Self-love empowers us to take risks and set boundaries for ourselves so that when we need to say no, we can. It also allows us to bounce back faster from setbacks and has a positive effect on our wellbeing, both physical and mental, as well as our relationships.

What I have found is that there are four parts to self-love.

Self-awareness is about knowing yourself: the things you like to do; what you don't like; knowing your values; boundaries; and what inspires you. Combined, they are what makes up you. Use a journal to write these aspects of yourself down and appreciate yourself for them.

Self-acceptance means loving all of you, regardless of any mistakes you make or successes you enjoy. Your mistakes are only miss-takes, so when you do them the next time, you have the chance to get them right.

Self-care is something many of us are not very good at. We are generally taught to care of others before ourselves. The truth is you need to take care of yourself before you think about other people. Create self-care habits that support your wellness; have some me-time doing what you love to do. Self-care is about investing in you.

Self-growth, I believe, is inherent in us. Each of us strives to be the best version of ourselves. The more we grow, the more fulfilled we are in our life.

Practising self-love goes beyond the surface. It takes both outer and inner work to understand our value and feel good about ourselves. To truly embrace it means to treat yourself the way you would like to be treated by others, accepting yourself for all of who you are so that you can be your own best friend.

How aware are you of your values?

Do you accept yourself for your mistakes and successes?

What is your favourite self-care ritual?

What self-growth work would you like to do?

"There is more wisdom in your body than in your deepest philosophy."

Friedrich Nietzsche

5

Understand your body

Ayurveda, otherwise known as The Science of Life, is an ancient healing system developed over thousands of years. In essence, its aim is to help you find balance and alignment with your true nature.

Within Ayurveda, there are three functional body types called your Prakruti which is your unique combination of the elements that make up your physical body, called doshas. They are Vata (air + ether), Pitta (fire + water), and Kapha (earth + water). Your Prakruti is set at birth and never changes throughout your life. Our body is made up of all the elements (air, ether, fire, water & earth) but dominant in two.

A Vata dosha is mostly air and ether and is the main driver of movement in the body including, heartbeat, respiration and contraction of muscles and also governs the nervous system. The physical qualities of someone with a dominant vata dosha are a thin frame, weak muscular system with dry skin and hair.

Their mental characteristics are they cannot stand still and perform activities fast. They are creative, learn fast and forgets just as quickly. They don't tolerate cold weather and prefer warmer food and drinks. When out of balance, they will have sleep or mood imbalances, occasional constipation, and mild aches.

The **Pitta** dosha is mostly fire and water and drives the digestion of food, maintains proper body temperature, comprehension of information, and gives colour and softness to the skin. They have a medium build and weight with thin hair and soft slightly moist skin.

Because pitta is sharp, oily, and hot, they benefit from cooling, heavy, dry foods with sweet, bitter, and astringent (beans, dried fruit apples, pears and pomegranates) tastes. If pitta is out of balance, they will become irritable and impatient, have occasional heartburn and acid reflux, skin rashes, acne, low blood sugar and find it difficult to fall asleep.

The **Kapha** dosha provides the structures and lubrication the body needs, and the stability to ground both the mind and body. People with dominant kapha will tend to have a large frame, gain weight easily and have thick oily hair and oily and moist skin. Their walk is slow but have excellent strength and endurance. They are calm and easy-going and don't like cold or damp weather.

Their digestion can be a little slow so they can easily miss a meal, they prefer dry food. You will know you are out of balance of you are depressed, fatigued, are gaining weight and suffering from coughs cold and congestion.

You will find Ayurveda and the doshas helpful in understanding how your body works, why you do the things the way you do, and why your partner may do them differently.

From that summary can you see which dosha you are?

Does it make sense to you now?

Do you understand your partner better?

If you would like to find out which dosha you are, go to the resources section at the end.

"You are needed in the world.
You were created on purpose and
with a purpose in mind."

Emily Gowor

6

Know your purpose

One of the regrets that people have on their deathbed is that they didn't do what they really loved to do. They did what was expected of them or what they thought they should do. They realise that what they had done didn't bring them joy, and they didn't feel fulfilled. So, at the end, it was just a job, and while they were maybe good at it, it didn't make their heart sing.

You might be one of those people in a 9-to-5 job that you have no passion for, and maybe you are questioning your purpose. What is my purpose and how do I find it? How will I know when I have found it? Do I even have to go to university? Isn't there someone already out there doing what I want to do?

Take my life, for example. I was one of seven children, and my father was a farmer. I went to a school with 23 other pupils, and then my father passed away from cancer when I was 10 years old. By the time I was 12, I was cooking for my mother and the three other siblings who were still living at home.

However, it wasn't until I was 65 that I found my purpose, which is nourishing and loving people through food. My life had already demonstrated what my purpose was, but I wasn't aware that it had until my daughter, Emily, created a purpose-finding tool to help people discover their true role in the world.

While your life journey will be completely different from mine, it will point and has been pointing you in the direction of your purpose. You just need some help to see what it is that you are on the planet to do this lifetime. My happy place is the kitchen where I create menus and create new dishes to tantalise people's taste buds.

If you haven't found your happy place yet, don't despair. What I want you to understand and take from this is that there is no one else like you on the planet. It doesn't matter if there are 1000 people who are doing what you are doing or want to do; not one of them have had the life you do.

It is the experiences we have that give us our wisdom. It gives us our perspective on our purpose. What is so important to remember is that there are people around the world who are seeking the answers to their problems that only you can solve. How amazing is that!

Once you know your purpose, then you can take the necessary steps to put it into action, whatever they may be and however long it takes. But rest assured, once you are in that place, you will be inspired from the inside, eager and excited to get out of bed and start each day.

Wishing you all the best!

What do you dream about?

What did you want to be as a child?

What has been a recurrent theme?

What is your happy place?

"*Trust the unfolding of your life; the universe has a plan far greater than you can imagine.*"

James Redfield

7

Live the life you dream of

Very few people are living the life they dream of. More often than not, people work in the same profession as their parents or they work in a job that they think they should do rather than one they enjoy. This pattern is sometimes repeated by our children and, in turn, our grandchildren.

Unfortunately, when growing up, children hear the word "No" many more times than "Yes" so that by the time they are out in the workforce, their unconscious automatically says "No" to the idea that you can do or be anything you want. So, any dream we may have had while growing up is slowly and surely snuffed out.

Rarely do people get a second chance at life, so unless you identify what is important to you in your career, relationships, and family and go after it, then you are likely to fall into the same trap with the same regrets and live a life of unfulfilled dreams.

It needs a total rewiring of our brain to realise that we can do what we want to do, and it is possible to love what we do. We are all looking to live a meaningful life. We want to feel fulfilled not only in our personal life but our professional life as well.

What is it that your friends say you do really well? What did you love doing when you were growing up? Doing what you love gives you the enthusiasm to keep learning new things, to expand your knowledge along with your skills.

People who love what they do naturally bring so much energy and productivity into their work through their passion. It is not just a job to them, and it won't feel like a chore. More importantly, you will be an inspiration to other people knowing that if you can do what you love, then they can too.

An amazing thing happens when you are doing what you truly love. The universe seems to line up the people you need and opportunities you are wanting with ease and grace and no effort on your part.

Fill your life with friends that help you level up, that inspire you and also want that for themselves. Spending time with negative people brings you down to their level rather than lifting you up to where you'd like to be.

The beautiful thing about living the life of your dreams is that you will feel that your life is complete and there is nothing else you want. You will know that you are getting the most out of your life, and so there will be no regrets.

After all my dear friends, life is a gift, so make the most of the one you have by doing what you love.

Go do it!

What are the things that you do well?

What is it you would love for your family?

How could you be less busy but more productive?

Do you know what your dream life looks like?

"Water is the most neglected nutrient in your diet, but one of the most vital."

Julia Child

8

Water, water, and more water

Although our body is made up of 60% to 80% water, we often miss or underestimate the importance of this fact. Water is the major component of all parts of our body with almost every bodily function relying on water.

Our body recognises a state of dehydration as a threat, causing anxiety. The amount of water we need varies from person to person depending on factors like our metabolism, the food we eat, and how active we are to the size of our body and the weather.

Water is a vital nutrient needed by our cells. It regulates our internal body temperature through sweat and respiration, lubricates our joints, and acts as a shock absorber for our brain and spinal cord, among other things. Water also helps to eliminate toxins and wastes from your body.

Lack of water causes the brain to not function normally and leads to difficulty in getting the chemicals to produce serotonin which regulates our moods. Research shows that once people are hydrated, they are calmer. Negative emotions like anger, confusion, tension, and fatigue decrease with hydration.

Because around 75% of brain tissue is water, dehydration reduces energy production in the brain and can change our brain structure, causing the brain to slow down. Serotonin, which stabilises mood and regulates our emotions, also cannot be produced. At the same time, this increases the production and release of the cortisol hormone, which increases our stress levels. At the molecular level, if water levels are too low, our brain cells cannot function properly, making the brain work harder to complete tasks.

Drinking fewer than two cups of water a day presents a greater risk of depression and anxiety, as there seems to be a correlation between the amount of water we drink and feeling depressed and anxious. Drinking less water may also influence how well you sleep.

It is much better to drink warm or hot water because it can be absorbed into the tissues more easily, while drinking cold water slows digestion down. Start your day off with a glass of warm water to help flush out the toxins that have accumulated during the night.

Do this after you have scraped the white toxic film off your tongue and finished oil pulling. Drinking a glass of warm water also cleanses your digestive tract, as well as increasing your metabolism ready to digest your breakfast.

Sipping water throughout the day is much better than swallowing a glassful at a time. Taking small sips allows your body to process the nutrients and makes it easier for your kidneys to process the fluid. Your kidneys filter over 189 litres of fluid a day and drinking plenty of water helps them do that more efficiently.

Cheers! (With water, naturally!)

How many glasses of water have you had today?

If you have a headache, it may be because you haven't had enough water.

What water are you drinking?

What container are you using for your water?

"If money colours everything, life loses its true meaning."

Emily Gowor

9
It's not all about the money

Of all the things people regretted at the end of their lives none – not one regret – was about money. We are so conditioned to the idea of money and what it allows us to do that we chase after it thinking it is the Holy Grail. But it isn't what gives our life meaning, and it is more likely to be one of the biggest worries that people have in their life.

You can reach your target savings, but unless you have a purpose for the money, you are left empty, without another goal to reach. Some people hit their goal and are then fearful that they might lose it. If you don't live your life according to your values, then having money for the sake of it is meaningless. It is almost a mirage, albeit a very shiny one!!

Wealth isn't as important as what it allows us to do with it. However, once you have all your needs met, then you are less dependent on material possessions and more focused on your social connections, your purpose, and the meaning of your life rather than it being about the money.

People who think that money will solve all their problems may be surprised and disappointed to find that when they have financial freedom, they still feel unfulfilled. The feeling of being content cannot be bought with money. Instead, it comes from having strong relationships, doing what you love, and building self-growth.

Of course, I'm not denying that a lack of money doesn't come with its own problems. A lack of money tells our brain that there is a threat to our survival, and as a result, influences the way a person thinks. At the end of the day, having enough money is just as important for our mental and physical wellbeing as it is for our financial freedom.

Rather than buying material things, it is time having experiences with people you love that provides lasting memories and opportunities for self-growth. What is best for you depends on what is meaningful to you and that which nurtures you on a deeper level. People can continually buy things that they think will make them happy, but it still leaves them empty and unsatisfied.

I think the truth is more likely to be that if you are content in yourself, then you don't need the money to make you happy – and if you are not content in yourself, then no amount of money is ever going to make you happy. Is this true for you?

Do you have left over at the end of the month?

Do you invest in shares?

Do you have a savings account for emergencies?

Will you have enough in your retirement fund?

"The most important thing about food labels is that you should avoid foods that have labels."

Dr Joel Fuhrman

10
Read the labels

*P*robably most of you don't worry about reading the food labels on packaged and canned food. Though if you want to eat cleaner food, then maybe it is time to stop and see just what is in the food you are buying. Manufacturers have tricky ways to label the same food.

Take sugar, for example. There is something ridiculous like 56 different names for sugar! This means you are probably buying a food that you think doesn't have much sugar, but there could be three or four different types of sugar in the product, just under different names.

Also, you are better off reading the labels on the back rather than believing any claims that have been made on the front of the packet. Those are there purely to lure you into buying the products by making health claims. Many processed products have "artificial flavours" listed as one of the ingredients.

These are chemical mixtures that resemble the flavour of an orange, apple, carrot, or whatever the flavour is supposed to be in the food. You will find them in many foods including baked goods, ice cream, snack foods, sauces, soft drinks, and lollies.

When you are grocery shopping, spend some time reading the list of ingredients because food labels can be confusing.

Perhaps it is wise to stay away from ingredients like artificial colours, natural flavours, aspartame, food colouring, guar gum and xanthan gum, all of which are made in a lab.

Other things to avoid are trans fats and over-processed oils like margarine, canola oil, palm oil, and hydrogenated vegetable oil which all increase inflammation and lower your good cholesterol.

At the end of the day, you want to be eating foods that your body recognises. You can eat healthy food without spending hours in the kitchen preparing it. But you do have to want to eat better. The saying goes that you are what you eat; I would rather say that are what you absorb. If you want lots of energy and mental clarity, the way to have those is by eating healthy food.

Reading labels can be time-consuming, complicated, and exhausting, but it is one of the most important things you can do to ensure that you are eating healthier and cleaner, especially once you understand the marketing tactics used to trick you into thinking you're eating healthy food.

You cannot raise your energy and attract positivity if all you're putting in your mouth is synthetic food that has little or no nutritional value – some of which you cannot even pronounce.

Do you take the time to read the labels?

Are you aware of the effects that some of these additives can have on your body?

Do you know what all the additives are?

Can you prepare the same food without additives?

"Perhaps the most significant thing a person can know about himself is to understand his own system of values. Almost everything we do is a reflection of our own personal value system. What do we mean by values? Our values are what we want out of life."

Jacque Fresco

11

Know your values

Our personal values are pivotal to who we are, who we want to be, and how we live our lives. When you live in your highest values, your life will be great. However, when you are not aligned, then life will feel more like a struggle. When you are aware of your highest values, you will use them to point you in the right direction to make the right choices.

Your values are likely to change during your life, although probably not dramatically. Take a moment and look at your life and the values that drive you. You might not have recognised that you have values, but you have been living according to them all your life.

Values are those characteristics that are important to you: family, for example. However, if you are working in a job six or seven days a week, then you are going to feel stressed and stretched because of the lack of time you can spend with your family.

You are putting work before family, which isn't in alignment with one of your core values. If this is the case, it may be a great idea to look at your values and see if you are living out of alignment with them.

My highest values are community, and, of course, food and love. They are intertwined. My love for food and my community are my values that have led me to choosing how I live my life today and is demonstrated in my daily actions.

When you look back through your life, look at the times when you felt confident, when everything was going well for you. Examine what was happening: who was in your life? What were you doing? What choices were you making? What factors contributed to you feeling confident and in control? What was happening when you felt the most fulfilled? What desire was being fulfilled? Why did these experiences give your life meaning?

When you have a list of your values, then it is time to prioritise them. Take two of them to begin with and compare them. If you had to choose between them, which value would you say is more important to you? Keep working through the list.

By comparing each value with every other value, you will eventually have your list of values in order from your highest to your lowest. Then, you could list strategies that would commit you to do things that are in line with your values.

Understanding your values and honouring them allows you to make informed decisions that will make your life easier and more fulfilling. It also helps you know yourself on a deeper level and you will be living the most authentic version of yourself. So, your values guide you back to who you truly are.

What do you think about most?

What do you love doing?

Do your values align with who you are?

Is there a value that you would like to take a higher place in your life?

"*Don't let anyone turn your sky into a ceiling.*"

Anonymous

12

Forget about what people think

At various times in our lives, I think most of us care what other people think; however, if you are a people pleaser – always needing external validation – then you may find that you will be doing things that are outside your values or may even not be in your best interests. It is far better for the validation to come from your inner self. Once you learn to love yourself, you won't need anyone's approval.

No one else but you can understand and appreciate the journey you have taken to get to this point in your life, so it is unreasonable for anyone to judge you or tell you what the best thing for you is to do.

Sometimes, though, parents have expectations for you to take a certain course of action, but in the end, it is only you who can decide if that is the right path for you. A fulfilling life isn't found by settling for one that is based on someone else's expectations.

Ultimately, no matter whether it is the opinions of your family or friends, they can only give you advice from their perspective, and that may or may not be the right advice for you at that time.

So, accept their advice, and then make the choice that is right for you. Those who don't fully share your reality can never appreciate the road you have been on to get to where you are right now. So, it is impossible for others to even think of telling you what you should or shouldn't do.

At times, a lot of us have issues with self-consciousness, where we lack the inner strength to be confident in making our own decisions. It is quite interesting that we live our lives wondering what others think of us, but, really, how much time do we think about other people's choices? They probably give so little time as you do to their choices because they are more focused on what they are doing rather than what you are doing.

It is more important for you to be authentic to yourself and make decisions from that place. You will have more confidence and self-esteem to be able to make the decisions that are right for you. You will attract like-minded people who appreciate you for who you are and what you are doing. Most importantly, they will support you along your journey.

Have courage and drop the false sense of who you think you are, who you think other people think you should be, what you think you ought to be, how you feel you need to behave, and you will be authentic.

I challenge you to make a decision and not think about what someone will think!

Are you able to decide without wondering what people will say?

What is the worst thing that could happen if you didn't get approval?

Whose approval do you need?

Do you have a self-image problem?

"Do what you love, and you won't have to work a day in your life."

Mark Twain

13
Do what you love

A regret many people had at the end of their life was that they didn't pursue their passion. They regretted spending so much of their time and effort on their job that they missed out on what really mattered.

They regretted that they didn't make their passion their work but, instead, worked in someone else's business. Some people had never even told anyone about their passion, and, for others, it was buried deep inside and never got the chance to be explored.

The truth is as a society we have become more concerned with having a 9-to-5 job that brings us money to support our family and buy a home. We aren't encouraged to explore our passions, much less even believe that we can do them. School, unfortunately, doesn't prepare young people for the rest of their lives, so as a result, teenagers leave school and if they don't go to university, they automatically get a job.

Reflect on what is your dream job and why it is your dream job. Are you doing that now or are you in a job that perhaps pays well but doesn't bring you joy? Does your current job leave you feeling fulfilled at the end of the day?

Doing what you love doesn't necessarily mean giving up everything – quitting your job to move to a beach somewhere to meditate every day – but what it does mean is that you can figure out what to pursue that makes you feel fulfilled and purposeful in life. It helps you make space for other areas of your life and not making work your whole life or its main purpose.

When you are doing the job you love, it will not only provide contentment, but it will also motivate you to do the best work possible, making you more productive. You won't need someone to motivate you to work to your potential or keep you accountable.

You will do your best work because you enjoy it. People who enjoy their work are more likely to learn faster, make fewer mistakes, be more optimistic, and ultimately make better business decisions.

The truth is that if you don't enjoy your work, then you will end up missing out on life and be one of those people who has regrets at the end of their life. It's not about working so much that it becomes your entire life. You need to be able to turn off from work and say, "OK, now I am going to spend time with my family or my hobbies."

Be honest and ask yourself, are you doing what you love?

Do you feel fulfilled?

Will you have regrets at the end of your life if you continue doing what you are doing now?

Do you spend enough time with your family?

"Getting all of the nutrients you need simply cannot be done without supplements."

Steven Gundry

14

Supplement your body

*I*n days gone by, our ancestors picked the food they were going to eat and ate it on the same day, gaining the full nutrients available in the food. Today, that isn't the case. In many instances, food is grown in another state or even another country and then it has to be transported many kilometres or across oceans to get to where we live. We are rarely growing our own food or eating locally, let alone eating seasonally (which I'll talk about later).

There are now so many of us on the planet that agriculture has had to change the way we grow crops, using more intensive practices and genetically modified seeds. Sadly, this has resulted in a reduction of the mineral content in the plants.

Mineral malnutrition is now considered to be the most serious global challenge to mankind in part because of the depletion of minerals like iron, zinc, selenium, and iodine in the food. These nutrients aren't replenished after the crop has been harvested because of poor management and the erosion of the topsoil, which contains most of the nutrients. Other deficiencies such as calcium, magnesium, and copper are also showing up in not only developing countries but developed countries as well.

A pivotal learning for me happened when I was listening to Vicki the Vego being interviewed on the radio. During the interview she said that three days after a lemon is picked, there is no vitamin C left in it. Vitamin C is water soluble, so it evaporates through the skin.

Therefore, it is probably safe to say that there is no vitamin C in any of the fruit and vegetables we buy from the supermarket or greengrocer, even in organic food, unless it is delivered by the farmer, and you buy it and eat it the same day or the next day.

So, to answer the question, do we need to take supplements to support our health? Yes, I believe that we do, especially if you are looking to fall pregnant, if you are ill and want to boost your immune system, or if you want to increase muscle. Below are my suggestions to start you on your supplement journey:

Vitamin D is important for bone health, mood, and metabolism. Because of the way we live now, very few of us spend enough time in the sunshine to get enough vitamin D.

Magnesium is needed for producing energy and promotes bone health.

Zinc supports our immune system.

Iron keeps our blood cells, energy, and brain function healthy.

Vitamin B12 creates and sustains our energy.

I suggest seeing an alternative wellness doctor and sourcing bloodwork, a gut microbiome test and even perhaps a hair test to safely identify which supplements you need and in which dosage, as, of course, our bodies are unique and so is our current state of health.

Do you take any supplements at the moment?

What do you feel is missing in your diet?

Are you always feeling tired?

Do you often fall ill?

"One cannot think well, love well, sleep well, if one has not dined well."

Virginia Woolf

15
The art of eating

The way we eat has changed radically over the years. At one time, we would have sat down at a table and enjoyed our meals as a family. Now, though, we are sitting at our computer mindlessly eating whatever we have in front of us, or we are eating while walking from place to place, or we are eating in front of the television. It is no wonder that so many people have gut issues not only from the food they eat but the way they eat.

Mindful eating allows you to become aware of your physical and emotional senses so that you can enjoy the food that you are putting into your body, really savouring its tastes and textures. You are more likely to chew your food longer compared to when you are mindlessly putting food into your mouth one bite after another.

You will also be more aware when you have had enough food, instead of eating everything on your plate just because it is there in front of you. When we are not eating mindfully, we miss the cue our body gives to say that we have had enough.

If you are feeling frustrated or angry or upset in any way before meals, take a few moments to transform your emotions before you begin eating. Give thanks for the food before you eat it and then enjoy the food, without any distractions.

Make a rule that there are no laptops, phones, or television while you are eating. Then you can be present for each mouthful and give it your full attention, which it deserves.

Experience your food with all your senses: sight, sound, taste, smell, and touch. Take in the flavours of each bite; put your knife and fork down between bites. Once you begin chewing your food, don't add more to your mouth.

The enzymes in your mouth go through a sequence. If you add more food to your mouth while chewing, some of the food won't begin the digestion process before it goes down to the stomach, most likely causing problems along the way.

Chew your food for as long as you can, preferably until there is no flavour left in the food. The more you chew the food, the less likely it will go through your body partly or largely undigested. It is important for you to know that when you eat while standing or walking, your body goes into flight or fight and actually shuts down your digestive process.

Do you chew your food until the taste is gone?

Are you conscious of the food in your mouth when you chew?

Do you eat when you feel upset?

Do you use your laptop while you were eating?

"The body benefits from movement, and the mind benefits from stillness."

Sakyong Mipham

16

Expand mindfulness

There are times in our lives when we are so busy that we have no time for anything else. Our heads are full of chitter-chatter as we go about our day-to-day work with no time to stop and be present — to smell the roses and allow new ideas to come to our minds or find solutions to the problems we face.

If you have ever driven somewhere and not remembered how you got there or walked into a room and forgotten what you went in there for, then it is probably time to become more present and mindful.

When you meditate or practise mindfulness, you empty your mind of its many thoughts. This allows you to be present to all that is around you, including the sights, the sounds, and smells that you were oblivious to previously. It allows you to be present with the people in your life, deepening your connections. The more order you have in your space and the more organised your time is (without being a perfectionist!) then the more mindful you will be.

Meditation and mindfulness can give you a more abundant, fuller, and meaningful life. You also adopt a sense of calm, peace, and balance that can benefit both your emotional wellbeing and your overall health. You can also use it to relax and cope with stress by refocusing your attention and increasing your awareness. It can help you learn to stay centred, to lower blood pressure, and improve your memory. It also can enhance your productivity as well as improve your performance.

You can become more mindful by giving your full attention to any of your normal daily activities. If your mind wanders, just gently allow the thought to pass without focusing on it, bringing your awareness back to the task at hand.

It allows you to tune in more deeply to anything you are experiencing. There are lots of moments when you can practise mindfulness during the day: standing in line at the supermarket, when you are washing the dishes, or even when you are going for a walk.

Maybe for your next meal, you can practise mindfulness. Be aware of the food on your fork as you put it in your mouth. As you are chewing, taste the different flavours, feel how your body responds.

If you haven't tried meditation, sit relaxed in a comfortable chair where there will be no distractions. Notice your breathing, in and out, and if your mind wanders, just refocus on your breathing. Even starting with just five minutes of meditation will help you feel more conscious and connected.

OK everyone, now close your eyes and take a deep breath in...

Do you find that your mind is full of chitter-chatter?

Are you able to sit still and clear your mind?

When you go for a walk, do you take your phone?

Try washing the dishes not thinking about anything but washing the dishes.

"We cannot become what we want by remaining what we are."

Max Depree

17

Start living today

*D*o you have regrets in your life? If you do, then don't wait until you are on your deathbed to evaluate how you've been living. Take the initiative today to make a change. Have the courage to see what your regrets are and use them to guide you in living the life you really want.

Most people on their deathbeds had not honoured even half of their dreams, and they died knowing that it was due to choices they had made or not made. It is a sad fact that most of us don't feel that we have the luxury of doing what we want in our life, and the most difficult regret to overcome is not doing what you love. This is why it is even more important to make the most of every day that we have.

To start living a meaningful life, the first step is to feel, have, and express love for yourself. Once you love yourself for who you are, you will become automatically dedicated and devoted to creating a life you truly love. You will give yourself permission to be who you truly are and pursue a career and personal life that fulfils you. It will also be easier to discover what your true purpose is – and then you can find a career that allows you to fulfil it.

To live fully, give up doing things that don't bring you joy or because your family or friends think you should. You are only going to be more stressed and unfulfilled, leading to regrets at the end of your life. Be present in your own life and on your own path.

Take a moment out of every day to reflect on the path you are on. Ask yourself: Is my path going towards an end goal that fulfils me? Or am I doing certain things because I feel I have to?

Perhaps the most important part of living this life you dream of is to fuel your body with nutritious food that has been cooked with love. Health brings freedom very few realise, until they no longer have it. Without your health, you can't fulfil your true potential nor realise your dreams. Nutritious food gives you the mental and physical energy to carry out your work each day and achieve the goals that have meaning for you.

I am not saying this is going to be easy, but it will be worth doing it. You will be less stressed, live longer, live without health problems, have a clearer mind, and feel content and fulfilled. Take it one step at a time. They say it takes three weeks for a habit to form, so try to take on one new habit every three weeks. It is the results from these small steps that will incrementally make a big difference in the coming years.

So, go forward with the confidence and courage to love deeply, follow your heart, dream big, and be kind to yourself.

Are you living your dream life?

Do you know what your dream life looks like?

Are you doing what you love every day?

Do you love yourself unconditionally?

"I have one rule, if you cannot eat it, don't put it on your skin."

Dr Saulius Alkaitis

18

If you can't eat it, don't put it on your skin

I used to go and listen to Don Tolman speak about food, health, and medicine among other topics. The main thing I remember him saying is that if you cannot eat what you are putting on your skin, then don't use it. This made so much sense to me and so, over time, I have stopped putting anything on my skin that I wouldn't put into my mouth.

The first thing I quit doing was using shampoo and conditioner. I guess that it was an easy task for the advertisers to tell people they needed both, and people fell for it: I fell for it! It took around three months before my hair felt natural and devoid of any residue of the conditioner.

It not only felt more natural, but it was so incredibly soft. Now, I treat my hair with coconut oil once a week, which strengthens my hair and leaves a seal of oil, adding protection and shine while keeping the moisture in.

You could use other oils like almond, grapeseed, or castor oil. I only wash my hair once a week because of my curly hair, and now that I am in the Vata stage of my life, my skin and hair are much drier, so I benefit from less washing. Naturally, I wouldn't be me if I didn't also mention that having a healthy diet will do a lot for your beautiful locks. I do suggest that if you are dying your hair then use dyes that are vegan.

As my skin becomes drier, I use aloe vera juice to nourish my skin, as well as heal any wounds from cuts to burns. Generally, I have found that if I continuously apply the aloe vera juice to any burn soon after it happens, then it leaves no scar. Aloe vera contains zinc, amino acids, and water, so it is great for moisturising skin.

For facial treatments, there are plenty of recipes online that use products like honey, coconut oil, oatmeal, and others. Maybe experiment and find something that you like. Some of the potentially harmful products are phthalates, formaldehyde, parabens, and oxybenzone, which you will also find in some sunscreen products.

Formaldehyde is used in the manufacture of clothing, especially cotton to control creasing, set colours so they last longer, and to prevent mildew, so it is important that you wash new clothes before you wear them.

I also make my own liquid soap and laundry liquid as well. Common ingredients in detergents will tend to include artificial fragrances, preservatives, carcinogens, allergens, surfactants, and chlorine bleach, any of which can be toxic.

If you can't eat it, don't put it on your skin

How many different products do you put on your skin?

Do you know what the ingredients are in each one?

Do you know the effects of each of the ingredients have on your health?

Do you wash your hair every day?

"*Intuition is seeing with the soul.*"

Dean Koontz

19

Listen to your intuition

*I*ntuition doesn't have anything to do with our mind or our thoughts. Intuitive thoughts happen so quickly that they don't even register with our conscious mind. We don't have to consciously think about it; we just know something is right or wrong.

Our intuition is different from having a gut feeling, which is a response to a fight or flight situation where we may find ourselves in a compromising situation and our instinct tells us to run.

Sometimes your intuition is as if there is another wise voice telling you what to do. It feels calm and grounded, a deep knowing. You don't have to reason it out, although the "hows" and "whys" may need to be worked out. Overthinking can sometimes challenge the results of your intuition since it might not make logical sense, but this is where you need to trust your intuition.

Intuition is the ability to know something without having to consciously think about it. Like the time you met someone, and all your senses went off like a siren letting you know not to interact with the person again. Another example of your intuition is when you are trying to solve a problem and because of the implicit knowledge you have stored, your intuition suddenly gives you the solution.

Have you ever had a nagging feeling that something just wasn't right, but you couldn't quite put your finger on it? Or maybe you've had a feeling about a decision you needed to make, but you listened to your intellect instead and then found that it didn't work out the way you wanted it to?

You can trust your intuition because it is a powerful tool that helps you make decisions that align with your innermost desires and values. Your intuition is a combination of your subconscious mind and past experiences which allow you to tap into a deep well of knowledge and wisdom that you may not be consciously aware of.

So, the next time you feel a strong hunch about something, don't be afraid to listen and trust your intuition. Usually, once you get used to listening to your intuition, you don't question whether it is right or wrong: you will just know that it is right.

Trusting your intuition can lead to better decision-making, increased self-confidence, and a stronger sense of purpose and direction in life. While it may not always be easy to follow your intuition, learning to trust it and rely on it can lead to a more fulfilling and authentic life.

The most important thing about your intuition is to not let your rational mind or the noise of others' opinions drown out your own inner voice and to have the courage to follow it.

What happened the last time you didn't follow your intuition?

Do you tend to allow your conscious mind to tell you to do something else?

Do you ignore any intuitive suggestions?

Do you trust your intuition?

"A recipe has no soul. You as the cook must bring soul to the recipe."

Thomas Keller

20

Put your soul into your cooking

My cooking experience began when I was 12 years old: I cooked because I had to. There was no choice for me. My mum was out in the dairy milking cows, and so it was left to me to cook dinner for me, my mum, and my three siblings who were still living at home.

It wasn't until I was in my 20s and cooking for friends that I realised I loved cooking. Not only did my friends enjoy the food I cooked, I did too, although I didn't understand why at the time!

When I owned a coffee shop in 2007 and 2008, the importance of loving your cooking was brought to my attention in the most interesting of ways. The customers coming to the café loved the food I prepared... however, they didn't enjoy my coffee. Yet they loved the coffee that my daughter, Cassie, would make for them.

Like most things, when you want to change, you need to be fully aware of what you are doing so you know what needs to change. So, I watched Cassie as she would make coffee for the customers, and I could see she was focused on the process. In contrast, when I prepared coffee, I was thinking about what I had to do next, what I needed to put on the shopping list, what the menu was for the next day – anything but the coffee. There was the answer to why my coffee was bitter.

When you are preparing food, be present! You want to love what you are doing. I believe that is why people mostly love their mum's cooking. Mums are not only present when they cook, but they love their children, and so the love often goes into the food.

A few years ago, I was cooking for a teacher who would come and pick her meals up on her way home from school. One night, she asked me what I did to the food she had the night before. I replied that I didn't think I had done anything differently, and I asked her why.

She said that as she was eating her meal, she would burst out laughing, but she didn't know what she was laughing at. Later that night, I recalled that while I was cooking her food, I was replaying in my head a comedy show I had watched. And so, while I was cooking, I was laughing at the memories, which she then picked up later in her food.

What I want you to understand from this is that what you are feeling when you are cooking will be experienced, felt, and received by the people who eat your food, whether that is anger, disappointment, hurt, stress, calmness, or love. So, why not cook with the love that you feel for the people you are cooking for!

What are you thinking about when you cook?

Have you ever had a coffee that tasted bitter?

Have you ever had a meal that was quite ordinary but tasted extraordinary?

Does your mum's cooking always taste great?

"Common sense and a sense of humour are the same thing, moving at different speeds. A sense of humour is just common sense, dancing."

Clive James

21

Keep your sense of humour

There is so much truth in the saying laughter is the best medicine. A sense of humour is one of the most important assets you can have as you grow older. It is a guard against taking yourself or life too seriously. It is also one of the best things you can do for your health and wellbeing. A healthy sense of humour keeps you light-hearted and helps you deal with adversity more easily.

There is no doubt that we are going through some of the toughest times most of us have ever known, both in our professional and our personal lives. It is no surprise that levels of mental wellbeing and human connections have all declined, especially since the beginning of Covid. However, that doesn't mean we should let our lives go by without laughing.

Laughter is said to have so many great health benefits, such as reducing stress and boosting the immune system. It can also be used as a tool in letting go of the emotions that you have after a challenging day at work. Humour and laughter are among the most valuable tools we have for strengthening bonds and relationships, diffusing stress, and tension, and raising our resilience.

Alas though, laughter is probably the last thing we think about when we are stressed. But let's face it, when we laugh, it is a challenge to feel anger, sadness, frustration, or anxiety. Laughter lowers the levels of the stress hormone cortisol and, surprisingly, increases your tolerance to pain.

There is no doubt that laughter relaxes us and triggers the release of endorphins, bringing joy into our lives as well as giving us an optimistic outlook. Laughter improves the function of blood vessels and increases blood flow, and it can also heighten our mood, bringing both our mind and body back into balance faster than the time it took to tell the joke. Laughter makes you feel good not just for a few minutes; the positive feelings remain with you long after the joke has been told.

Seeing the funny side of something that happened can give a different perspective and enable you to move forward without feeling bitter or resentful.

Who knows, maybe laughing helps you live longer, or you might even burn extra calories? What I do know for sure is that laughter makes life more fun and enjoyable, especially when everything feels a bit too serious. Do you know the joke about the giraffe that took three months to get over a cold?

How many times have you laughed today?

Who or what makes you laugh?

Are you able to see the funny side of a serious situation?

Maybe you could try laughter yoga at a YouTube near you!

*"If you're healthy,
you're wealthy."*

Yiddish Proverb

22
Live your healthiest life

G ood health can offer many benefits, but it is one of the biggest challenges we face.

Today, in the midst of all the hustle and bustle of daily life, especially since Covid, one of the outcomes is that maintaining a healthy lifestyle has become a problem for a lot of us. We became a society that found it easier to order a takeaway meal instead of cooking for ourselves.

We couldn't go out and spend time enjoying the benefits of nature, and so many of us now don't go out as much as we used to. For some of us it has been challenging making time for friends and loved ones. We have become addicted to social media, spending more time alone, on our phones and laptops.

All this leads to stress and health problems that you often ignore in your day-to-day routine, until one day, you are forced to be still by an illness or broken bone. It is much better for you to prevent that from happening and maintaining a healthy lifestyle by keeping fit and free of illness.

Good health gives you the strength and energy to help you achieve better results in every aspect of your life. Being able to sleep at night, walk without pain, eat, and enjoy food is the main meaning of contentment.

Your overall health and wellbeing, including your emotional, mental, spiritual, and physical health, should always be your number one priority. So, start making the following a part of your daily routine.

Eat a healthy breakfast every morning. People who eat a good breakfast are less likely to overeat the rest of the day. Drink plenty of water: your body needs it to maintain a fluid balance and to transport nutrients throughout your body, help in digestion, and control body temperature. Get a good night's sleep.

Find ways to lessen stress by connecting with friends, managing your time more effectively, walking in nature, and spending time doing what you love. Turn problems into opportunities with positive thinking and lower your blood pressure, improve your immune system, and gain confidence. Eat a well-balanced healthy diet with more whole grains, fruit, and vegetables, while limiting intake of high-fat and refined sugar foods.

I wouldn't expect you to try and take on all these suggestions at once, so take one at a time. Adjust things to suit you and see how you go, acknowledging that it does take time and you may have setbacks. Be kind to yourself if you do experience the odd setback.

What areas of your health do you think you could improve?

Do you need to increase your exercise?

What parts of your diet could be better?

What is the level of stress in your life?

"If you keep learning and trying new things, meeting new people, your life will always be interesting and fun."

Mama Rae

23
Learn new things every day

Luckily for me, learning is one of my highest values. I have always been curious, needing to know about everything around me and how it works. That hasn't changed during all the years of my life. I still have the insatiable 'need to know' I had as a child.

Let's face it, there is so much to learn and know. I believe that it is one of the reasons I am open-minded and why I find joy in everything around me. My life is so much richer.

Studies have shown that learning new things can improve your memory, cognitive abilities, and mental wellbeing. Learning can also prevent or delay the onset of dementia and Alzheimer's disease.

Learning keeps your mind sharp, stimulating new neural connections while strengthening existing ones. It can enhance creativity by being open to new ideas, motivating you to learn more as well as stimulating your curiosity, which can lead to innovation and better problem-solving skills.

It improves your memory and attention span. It expands your horizons in lots of ways, bringing joy and meaning to your life. Learning helps you acquire new skills and knowledge that can make you more employable and adaptable in a changing world. It fosters a lifelong habit of curiosity and exploration, which can keep you mentally active and engaged, challenging you to grow and improve yourself, boosting your confidence. It also makes you happier and more fulfilled.

Learning increases your knowledge and, hopefully, wisdom, empowering you to make informed decisions and to take action, which can have a positive impact on yourself and others. It enhances your communication and critical thinking skills, which can help you express yourself and understand others better.

Being curious about and then seeking new information exposes you to new ideas and perspectives that enrich your worldview and your life. It gives you a sense of accomplishment, boosts your self-esteem and sparks your curiosity and creativity, and makes not only life, but you, more interesting.

So, hands up: Who is up for learning something new today?

What have you learned today?

What would you like to learn about?

Do you make time to learn new things?

What would it take for you to want to learn something new?

"Quit eating sugar. If you make one change to improve your gut health, make it this. Bad bacteria love sugar and feed off it."

Dave Asprey

24
Break your sugar addiction

When I decided to remove refined sugar from my diet, I was amazed at just how much sweetness was in the food without adding more sugar to it. There is natural sweetness in so many foods that I can make a cheesecake with less than a quarter cup of maple syrup. It also allows you to taste the flavour of the other ingredients, rather than having them masked by the sugar taste.

Sweet is one of the six tastes, (together with salty, sour, bitter, astringent, and pungent) and it is found naturally in foods with nourishing macronutrients like fats, proteins, and carbohydrates; it is also used by our body to build muscle or fat tissue. If you are getting enough sweetness from your food, your body won't crave more sugar.

Sugars are prevalent in the food processing industry because they bulk up the product and add flavour. They are also used as a preservative and a thickener. Unfortunately, there are around 56 different types of sugar used in the processing process, and many are disguised under different names, with many products containing more than one type of sugar.

A high-sugar diet can lead to many diseases including high blood pressure, increased cholesterol levels, inflammation, insulin resistance, obesity, and type 2 diabetes. Fructose, which is found naturally in fruits, corn syrup, and table sugar, acts negatively on the leptin hormones that tell your brain when you have eaten enough.

So, a high-fructose diet can you leave you feeling hungry even when you have overeaten. An excess of sweet foods, especially refined sugars and grains, thickens your blood plasma which causes high blood pressure and poor circulation.

If you have a high sugar intake and would like to do something about it, try a detox tea of 1 teaspoon each of cumin, coriander, and fennel seeds. Add those to 1 litre of boiling water and simmer for 10 minutes. Sip it throughout the day, finishing before 5:00pm. It resets your palate, and you will find that the sugar craving will disappear in as little as a week, although it may take a few months if your diet is very high in sugar.

Honey and fruits may be a safe way to satisfy your sweet cravings without causing weight gain and blood sugar problems, and they are also much less addictive. Raw honey is a great natural fat metaboliser and stabilises blood sugar, and its warming quality boosts your energy. Choose sweet foods that also have some fibre in them as they keep blood sugar more stable.

Are you aware of how much sugar you are drinking and eating?

Are you aware of the sugar content in the processed foods and drinks you have?

Are you showing signs of having pre-diabetes?

Try eating foods that have natural sugar in them.

"A walk in nature walks the soul back home."

Mary Davis

25

Appreciate nature's gifts

Many of us spend most of our time indoors or in transport to and from work, which means we spend very little time outdoors. Our weekends are spent doing household chores, shopping, and washing, which means we are missing out on the benefits that nature can give us, not only from the physical but also from the mental aspect.

Being in nature can take us out of our heads and just allows us to be present with all that is around us: the wind whispering through the trees; the sound of the birds chirping; the beautiful smells in the air from the wet grass.

There is something about the restful calm of nature that is transformative, which, for me, is almost instantaneous. The moment I step on the grass, I feel in a tranquil place. It is so easy to leave my thoughts behind and clear my head, let go of the stresses, just relax, and enjoy mother nature. I know that I will sleep much deeper after a walk in the park or along the river during the day.

There are so many benefits to spending time in nature, especially for our mental health. It allows us to be more present, gives us clearer focus, and often it gives you a fresh take on what is happening in your life. The colours, patterns, and shapes found in nature ignite our imagination and creativity; I often get ideas for my paintings when I am in the park.

Being outside can be motivation to do it more often, helping you stay fitter and more active. It has been scientifically proven that experiencing a walk through the park, sitting by a river, or lying in the sun lowers stress and promotes wellbeing.

Let's face it, we could all do with more time in the sunshine soaking up Vitamin D. Because we spend so much time indoors out of the sun, most people are most likely deficient in this important vitamin.

On a physical level, time in nature can do many things like lower your heart rate, tension in your body can be released, and your cortisol levels can lessen. Even taking your shoes off and grounding yourself to the earth is like recharging your positive energy, bringing a change in your mood with it.

The next time you sit down in front of the TV to watch a movie, think instead of going out to enjoy Mother Nature where you can slow down and connect more with yourself free from any distractions. Take some deep breaths, clear your mind, and become aware of the sights and sounds around you. Just absorb them, without thinking about it. How do you feel now?

How often do you spend time outdoors?

When was the last time you went for a walk without your phone?

Where is your favourite place?

Do you make it a regular practice?

"Exercise is King, nutrition is Queen: put them together and you've got a kingdom."

Jack LaLanne

26

On your bike and exercise!

Overall, a lot of people are probably moving less than they did before Covid, sitting behind a screen for longer periods of time than ever before. Exercise could be declared preventative medicine if you want to have a healthy lifestyle. The benefits of exercise are many and include boosting energy, maintaining your weight, building strength, and preventing health problems from arising.

Exercise can also help you to lose weight, and it helps ease pressure on your joints, ligaments, and tendons, making them more flexible. Better flexibility and mobility can make it easier to move around and may decrease your chance of falling because it helps with balance. You sleep better too! Having a good rest is important to both your mental and physical health: it improves your concentration and gives you more energy.

If you find it challenging to exercise, then ask a friend to do it with you. It helps to have an accountability partner to keep each other motivated and on track. Exercise can also reduce your cholesterol levels and improve cardiovascular fitness. Of course, a healthy diet is just as important. (You knew that was coming, didn't you?!) Truly though, eating well will give you the energy to exercise.

Exercise also benefits your mental health by reducing anxiety, depression, and any negative moods by improving your self-esteem and cognitive function. If you are suffering from social withdrawal, you could try going for a walk every day. Being active increases the level of endorphins in your body which puts you in a better mood. As you realise how much exercise you have done as time passes, it will increase your self-esteem and confidence as well.

A sedentary lifestyle on the other hand leads to the risk of heart disease, diabetes, high blood pressure, obesity, and osteoporosis. So, no matter how old you are, it is never too late to start exercising. It doesn't have to be scary.

Aerobic exercises can be swimming, cycling, jogging, walking, gardening, or maybe even dancing. Choose something that you like doing. Remember, it isn't necessary to exercise every day; you can go for a brisk walk three times a week and still get benefits. Try starting small and build up as you get into the rhythm of the exercise you choose.

You will find that exercising will increase your overall health and wellbeing, so why not start today?

On your bike and exercise!

How much exercise are you doing daily?

Are you raising your heart rate for part of your exercise?

How can you make time to exercise?

What excuses do you make for why you don't exercise?

"You can choose courage, or
you can choose comfort.
You cannot have both."

Brené Brown

27

Live boldly

Most of us are set in our ways going about our everyday normal activities. We become so familiar with our routine that it is easy to stay in that place where it is comfortable – there is no anxiety, you feel at ease, and you don't need to push the boundaries. You can just stay in your safety bubble. It doesn't create any apprehension or stress. But the problem is, it isn't a place: it is a feeling, a feeling of safety and familiarity.

Imagine who you would be if you did get out of your comfort zone. Take a moment and look back on your life and the times when you embraced doing something for the first time: your first day at high school; your first date or your first driving lesson.

All these actions needed you to go into the unknown. Without getting out of your comfort zone how can you grow and move forward? You can miss the amazing opportunities that are there waiting for you.

I am sure you know what it is like on a wet Saturday afternoon when you are bored and suddenly get a bright idea. Well, my bright idea was to dye my hair – only, it didn't quite turn out as well as I would have liked. It was so dark I felt like I was me but in somebody else's body! I persisted with it, until one day I noticed a sign on the hill advertising the *Be Brave*

Shave campaign for childhood cancer. I thought to myself, there is my solution.

Without thinking about the consequences, I made an appointment. It wasn't until I sat in the chair that I realised I was out of my comfort zone. Unexpectedly, my discomfort extended way beyond the shave, which I wasn't prepared for. For several weeks people wouldn't look me in the eye, obviously thinking I had cancer. It felt so isolating but at the same time I felt so much compassion for the people who had cancer.

The fact is, though, being out of your comfort zone brings so many rewards. It allows you to grow and, really, isn't that what we are all looking to do, to be a better version of ourselves? By pushing through your personal boundaries, you will find the courage and the confidence to take on anything.

It is said that life begins when you try something new. So next time you are on the edge of your comfort zone, remember that by taking the plunge you will remove some of the fear and you will become more empowered.

What happened when you were taken out of your comfort zone?

Do you fear taking risks?

What is the worst that could happen?

What is the best thing that ever happened to you when you were living boldly?

"The longer I live, the more beautiful life becomes."

Frank Lloyd Wright

28

Age the way you want

Aging is an attitude as much as it is a physical process. Just like anything in life, you can choose to be healthy, vibrant, and joyful as you age, or you can be bored and unfulfilled and live your life with your doctor as your best friend. It is all about the choices you make.

My desire to live an active, healthy, and joyful life was set when my father passed away from cancer of the bladder. The last ten months of his life were spent in hospital receiving treatment and immersed in pain. As a 10-year-old, it was painfully challenging to watch my dad decline from the vibrant, energetic man I knew to the one laying in a hospital bed waiting to die.

So, as I grew older and learned more about health and sickness, I consciously made the choice to live my life not only free of illness but with love, passion, and fun. To this point, I am on track.

I haven't been ill nor needed to see a doctor for 36 years. I don't take any medications, and I don't wear glasses. In fact, someone asked for some aspirin recently and I had to say that I don't keep any in the house.

My life since my dad's passing has all been leading up to where I am right now, from the close attention to my diet, the continual learning, seeing the magic around me, hosting dinner parties for friends, the love I have for people, to sharing my life's wisdom with you within this book. I feel such gratitude for everything that has happened in my life and to the people I have met.

It is interesting to note that the world-famous architect Frank Llyod Wright is known for having done his best work in the later years of his life, from his 60s until his death at 92. This proves beyond any doubt that you can contribute to society in a meaningful way, even if you aren't an architect, for a long time after what we consider to be the retirement age.

We don't have to buy into the cultural expectation of what any age should be like or feel like or even act like. In fact, I have decided that I won't be 75 years old in April (the month that this book launches to the world), but I will have reached level 75 instead.

I have wonderful friends of all ages who love me as I am. So, I can be me, without worrying about how I am dressed, what I say or do or what shenanigans I get up to. It is a blessing to be able to do that without worrying what people are going to say.

What if instead, you could consciously level up, accepting yourself for who you are and the level you are at and define your own path? You could then look forward to levelling up with joyous anticipation!

What level are you at?

What could you do to bring more joy into your life?

What is your favourite hobby?

Do you have friends you can call on?

"It's difficult to think anything but pleasant thoughts while eating a homegrown tomato."

Lewis Grizzard

29

Fresh is best

There are two schools of thought about how long you should keep any food that is left over from your meals. According to science, leftover food can be eaten three or four days after it has been cooked, although there are conditions to that, including how the food is stored, how long it has been left before being refrigerated, how it is defrosted, and how hot the food is when you are reheating it.

If you know you won't eat the food within three to four days, then put it in the freezer where it will keep for a long time, but it will taste best if eaten within three months.

After three days in the refrigerator, the likelihood of bacteria growing in the food increases the risk of food poisoning. Though the look, smell, or taste of the food won't be any different. So, if you are concerned at all, then the saying, "If in doubt, throw it out," applies here.

Cooked food needs to be refrigerated within an hour. The key to food safety is to keep hot food hot and cold food cold and to minimise the amount of time it is in the danger zone, which is from 4°C and 60°C, which is when bacteria can multiply fast.

Then there is the second school of thought, Ayurveda, which incorporates medicinal and nutritional value and follows that the longer food stands after it has been cooked, the less nutritional value it has. The medicinal value of essential oils and the breakdown of unique phytochemicals is fast, while the nutritional value of the food mostly happens more slowly.

Raw food after it is picked is alive and has all the nutrients in it until it is cooked, when the nutrients then die. As it decomposes, so do the nutrients and phytochemicals. Also, exposure to heat and light reduces the nutritional value of the food.

Any leftover food you reheat will remove more of the nutritional value, especially heat-sensitive vitamins like vitamin C and the B vitamins. If your digestion isn't as strong as it could be, then may find that after eating left-over food that is more than 24 hours old will leave you suffering from bloating and flatulence. The next time you eat left-over food that is more than a day old, take notice if you feel bloated after your meal!

It is worth remembering that not all bacteria that is in the food you left out overnight are killed in the reheating process, even at high temperatures. Seventy years ago, food could be left out and eaten the next day without having any problems but because pathogens are more virulent today eating food that has been left out overnight is not recommended.

Do you have flatulence when you have eaten food that is two to three days old?

Do you experience bloating after eating your meal?

Do you eat food that you cannot remember when you cooked it?

Do you reheat food in the microwave hot enough to kill any bacteria?

"By cleansing your body on a regular basis and eliminating as many toxins as possible from your environment, your body can begin to heal itself, prevent disease, and become stronger and more resilient than you ever dreamed possible!"

Hippocrates

30

Reduce your toxin intake

In the world we live in today, we cannot escape toxins. They are in our food, the air we breathe, and in the environment. On average we are exposed to over 700,000 different toxins every day, from cosmetic products and plastic water bottles to cleaning products which all contain chemicals that may not be good for your health.

While our body has a natural detoxing system, we need to help our bodies by minimising toxins on top of helping to eliminate them. Small amounts of toxins may go unnoticed; however, once your body reaches a tipping point, then you can have some unpleasant side effects such as brain fog, bad breath, weight gain, nausea, and fatigue.

Many chemicals are toxic because they poison the enzymes which are necessary for every physiological function in your body, including lowering your protection against oxidative stress. They also prevent the production of haemoglobin in your blood which carries oxygen around your body. Your body cannot then function properly, which can lead to diseases like cardiovascular, cancer, and Parkinson's.

While you can limit your exposure to toxins, it's impossible to remove your exposure altogether. However, there are things that you can do to lower your intake of toxins. One important thing I tell people is to wash any new clothes you buy before you wear them. There are around 6000 different synthetic chemicals used in the production of clothes, including formaldehyde and chlorine bleach.

If you happen to scratch the surface of your non-stick frying pan, then you are exposing you and your loved ones to toxic substances. It is time to throw it out. When you are out and about and need water, it is best if you use a copper or glass drinking bottle rather than a plastic bottle.

It isn't easy but do your best to limit your toxin intake. Make sure your diet is clean and healthy and that your gut is digesting your food so that you are hungry at the next mealtime. If you aren't hungry, then it means you still have food in your stomach which hasn't been digested.

There are things you can do to increase your digestive fire so that you are hungry at mealtime: eat three meals a day, at the same time each day; make lunch your biggest meal of the day; eat dinner before 7pm; make sure your drinks are at room temperature or warmer – remember that cold food or drink slows down your digestion. Don't work and eat, but sit, relax, and eat mindfully.

Do you drink water from plastic bottles?

Has the surface of your non-stick frying pan been scratched?

What is your digestive fire like?

How could you improve your diet?

"*I love you not only for what you are, but for what I am when I am with you.*
I love you not only for what you have made of yourself, but for what you are making of me.
I love you for the part of me that you bring out."

Elizabeth Barrett Browning

31

Tell your nearest and dearest you love them

One of the greatest regrets of people on their deathbed is that they didn't tell their loved ones how much they meant to them, which is so sad. We all want to feel loved, wanted, and needed by the people close to us. In other words, people get so caught up in the day-to-day busyness of life that they put off doing the things that are truly meaningful to them.

When you take the future for granted, it's easy to lose sight of larger questions of meaning and purpose and respond to what's demanding your attention in the moment.

While some of us readily say "I love you" to our loved ones, not everyone is able to openly express their love. We all have our love language, using either touch, words of affirmation, acts of service, quality time with our family, or we give gifts to the ones we care about.

My mother had a different love language from me, but as a child, I didn't understand, so, naturally, I thought that she just didn't love me. However, when I understood that her way of saying "I love you" was through acts of service, it all made sense.

After riding the three kilometres home from school on a cold winter's day, my dear mum would have a pot of hot soup on the stove for us. That was how she showed her love for us.

Looking back, I can see that I tested the boundaries in almost all ways I possibly could to get attention from my mum because I didn't have the secure attachment to her that I needed to grow my self-worth and emotional intelligence.

The presence of a love language is considered crucial because it can help you and your loved ones understand each other better and with greater depth. A love language is the way our love is expressed in the form of actions, behaviours, and attitudes that make a person feel valued and loved.

It shows we care about them, which can help strengthen relationships and help us understand each other's needs and desires. Knowing the type of love language that the person you care about has is important because it means you can express sincere feelings of affection and love for that person and know that they received it deeply.

Love is all that truly matters. You must tell the people you love that you love them. It can feel uncomfortable or vulnerable at times, and you might say to yourself, "Oh, they know," ... but people need to hear it!

When is the last time you told someone you loved them?

When did you last tell yourself how amazing you are?

Do you know your partner's love language?

Can you identify your parents' love language?

"When you catch a glimpse of your potential, that's when passion is born."

Zig Ziglar

32

Be all of who you are

The truth is we have the possibility to not only be who we want to be but also do anything we want to do. When we are born, we are like a piece of clay ready to be moulded any way we like.

It is interesting that as children we do feel that we can do anything and be anyone we want to, until a time comes when, as teenagers, we lose our self-esteem and confidence, and we do or say things that aren't really who we are just so that we fit in.

The need to fit in becomes an unconscious part of how we speak and act and as an adult. The 'real' world takes over, and we continue to do whatever we need to do without ever questioning what it is we want to do or who we want to be.

We mould ourselves to fit in to society's bubble of go to work; earn money; go to work; earn money. If we are lucky, we get to enjoy the money sometimes. Mostly though, people are on the treadmill of life, and don't ever get off that treadmill. I guess that is one reason why so many people have all those regrets at the end of their life, which I find sad and unfortunate.

We are all born with a genius inside, but so few of us even get to know their genius much less get to use it. Apart from that, the world never gets to experience or benefit from all of our genius that lays dormant.

When you know yourself deeply, you are more likely to experience a fulfilling and rewarding life, otherwise you are likely to end up conforming to society's values and losing touch with who you are. I believe that it doesn't necessarily take as much courage to remain true to yourself, even with all the distractions and influences of social media and society in general when you have a good sense of self.

When you are comfortable with the real you and have a strong sense of identity, you will always be able to come back to you, even with all the distractions or when you are feeling lost.

Live up to your own aspirations, not down to others' expectations. There is no passion to be found in settling for a life that is less than the one you are capable of living.

So, be courageous and get out of your comfort zone or your boring job, discover what you are here to do and be, and develop and share your own unique gifts and talents with the world that I know is out there waiting for you. You can do it!

Do you express your uniqueness?

Do you know what your genius is?

Are you clear about what you are on the planet to do?

Are you being all of who you are in the world?

"Magic exists. Who can doubt it, when there are rainbows and wildflowers, the music of the wind and the silence of the stars?"

Nora Roberts

33

See the magic around you

*I*t is incredibly sad to see people today walking along the street with their eyes glued to their phones or seeing two people sitting together in a café, both using their phones, oblivious to what is going on around them. The universe has a lot to teach us, but we can only learn if we are open and willing to look beyond what is happening on the screens in front of us.

Finding magic in life is all about noticing the little things and appreciating everything there is. It will change your perception and your senses will become more acute. It can be as simple as the beautiful colours of the sunset, the rainbow that suddenly appears, or the spontaneous giggle of a child.

The magic that is happening around us can give us inspiration for solutions to problems we want to solve. Sometimes the solution comes when we are not thinking about it but when our mind is clear.

One morning, when my two youngest children were three and four years old, we were in the garden and I showed them the cap on the Californian poppy plant coming off the bud, allowing the flower to open fully. They were both so mesmerised and fascinated that each morning after that magical experience, we were in the garden again waiting to see if there were any caps ready to come off the buds. That's the magic of nature!

It is unfortunate that when we grow into adults, we tend to lose the ability to see the magic around us as we become so engrossed in the expectations of being an adult. We find ourselves stuck in a job that doesn't bring us joy and makes us feel empty, living a life that is meaningless.

Many of us become so burned out and suffering with mental health issues that we have forgotten that child-like fascination with all things magical and what it does for our wellbeing. How can one be depressed when we see something magical that lifts us up?

This planet is full of magical things. The stars in the night sky, the fish jumping in a babbling brook, three rainbows simultaneously over the hills, the sunlight shining through the trees, and people laughing on the street.

To see this magic, you need to be aware of what is happening around you. Meditation or mindfulness and putting your phone away will allow you to be in the present moment so that you can see and appreciate what magic is there right in front of you.

When was the last time you sat outside at night and marvelled at the stars in the sky?

When did you last stand in the park and smell the freshness after the rain?

When was the last time you watched a sunrise or sunset?

Have you noticed the way the light shines through the trees?

"Eat only when you feel hungry.
Notice and feel your hunger.
This is conscious eating."

Deepak Chopra

34

Eat when you are hungry

There is hunger and then there is appetite. Hunger is the body demanding nutrients so it can function normally. Appetite, on the other hand, is when you have eaten a large dinner and then decide you can eat some dessert as well, whether you need it or not. The dessert looks so good you cannot say no.

Appetite isn't true hunger: it is a desire to eat. It comes on fast and is often caused by emotional or environmental factors as well. Our lifestyle provides numerous triggers for your appetite to be satiated.

Packaging is very attractive, the snack foods are at eye height in the supermarket, and, of course, the cooking shows on TV. Unfortunately, we were all programmed to eat all the food on our plate as children, and we have never learned to recognise when our stomachs were full.

We also respond to our emotions by eating. Whether we are bored, sad, disappointed, angry, stressed, or excited, we generally enjoy eating snacks and foods that are high in salt and sugar. Then there are the social occasions when we all are probably guilty of eating too much.

Some people have other habits when they are working at home in front of their computers while eating their meals at the same time. Apart from not even being aware of what they are eating, they have no idea when they are full and so will more than likely overeat.

If you happen to be bored, stressed, or upset and you see food that smells delicious, it can increase your appetite even if you aren't hungry. The problem with eating when you aren't hungry is that you can start to put on weight and feel mentally dazed and heavy. Whereas a delicious and nutritious meal when you are hungry can give you both physical and mental energy.

Real hunger is different in that it comes on slowly, so you can put off eating for a while, but you cannot ignore it. You could also look at the triggers that cause you to eat when you aren't hungry and find healthy outlets for your emotions, like listening to music or meditating or going for a walk.

If you are someone who eats your meals at the same time each day, check to see whether you are hungry or not – it could be because it is your routine, or it could be more from appetite rather than hunger.

For most people it is the small things they do every day that are the biggest problem, not the once-a-week treat!

Do you eat at the same time every day?

Have you noticed whether you are hungry or not at mealtimes?

When you feel hungry it means your digestion is working.

Have you tried checking if you are thirsty rather than hungry?

"If you ever start taking yourself too seriously, just remember, that we are talking monkeys on an organic spaceship flying through the universe."

Joe Rogan

35

Don't take yourself seriously

We take ourselves too seriously by needing to control things that we mostly have no control over. Most of us at times fall back into being serious when we are stressed or overwhelmed or when things don't go to plan, especially in the busyness of the world as it is today. Some of us spend too much time sweating over the small stuff.

I'm not saying that we should never be serious. Of course, there are times when seriousness is called for – when we are planning our future, our goals, or when we are with the bank manager – then we totally need to be serious.

Not taking yourself seriously is being able to accept yourself and most of the things happening around you as not life-threatening. Most of the time these things shouldn't even concern you because it is just part of what happens from time to time in the world.

But when you live from day-to-day anxious and uptight, you are not allowing enough fun and spontaneity into your life so that it becomes enjoyable. If it is challenging for you to look at the situation and be able to see the funny side, then you are taking yourself much too seriously.

It's great to be ambitious and have expectations, but if you are too focused on your goals that you don't take the time to acknowledge yourself for how far you have come, then you are being too serious. If you find yourself feeling like this, then it is probably time to take a step back, loosen up, and see what you have achieved.

Maybe you have just spoken on a stage to a large audience, and when you have finished people congratulated you on your presentation; however, you can only think of all the things you didn't say that you would have liked to have said to the point that you cannot accept the compliments.

That, my friend, is taking yourself too seriously. It is impossible to be perfect all the time. Things happen that jeopardise our plans, so embrace your perfectly imperfect human self and release the unnecessary pressure of living up to your high expectations.

The fact is change is inevitable; your parents pass; your children grow up and leave home; things don't always go as you planned. Life is not always a bed of roses. The more you loosen up and accept that life isn't structured and orderly, the more you open the space for change, play, fun, and so much more.

Do you like everything to be perfect all of the time?

What do you say to yourself if you make a mistake, or something doesn't go as planned?

Are you able to see the humorous side of your mistakes?

When was the last time you had a walk in the park?

"If you see someone without a smile, give them one of yours."

Dolly Parton

36
Smiles make the world a better place

*E*ven if you have to fake it at first, smiling a little will cause your brain to start releasing the feel-good hormones that leave you with a genuine smile on your face. If you are not having a particularly good day, smiling will soon lift your mood, as well as the moods of the people you smile at.

Smiling can lower your blood pressure; it makes you more attractive to others, and it reduces your stress. All that is good for your overall wellbeing. I feel that the more you smile at people, the more you want to smile. Try it for yourself! Smiling is one of the best things you can do for your health and wellbeing because it can boost your immune system and make you feel better.

The best thing about a smile is it is contagious. Most people you send a smile their way will smile back. Who knows? It may be the only smile they get all day! It is almost like we are hard-wired to smile. There is also a ripple effect that your smile can have, especially if the person you smiled at wasn't having a particularly fun day. You never know what is going on in another person's life, but a smile could completely transform their day.

I tend to smile at almost everyone when I am shopping, regardless of whether I know them or not. I have noticed some of them when they see me another day will smile at me first, like they remembered me.

I expect that smiling makes you look confident and more approachable, and we tend to bond with people who make us feel like that. When someone smiles at us, there is a sense of feeling fulfilled and content. When you smile at someone you know, you are communicating to them that you see and appreciate them.

Just as stress permeates our entire body, the effect of smiling loosens tension your body. Smiling relaxes the muscles in your face, which helps to tone your facial muscles and increase the blood flow, improving your complexion, and making you look younger. And don't we all want that?

Another great reason to smile is that, apparently, it extends your lifespan, so surely that is reason enough to smile. Smiley people are also more likely to enjoy better health. It is not that much of a stretch of the imagination to see that smiling is part of living a healthy lifestyle.

Go on, I dare you to smile!

Next time life is a little challenging, why not try smiling your way out of it?

Try smiling today at someone you don't know.

In fact, smile at a lot of people. How does your mood change?

Try smiling, just because you can!

"The finest thing about a hobby is that you can't do any pretending about it. You either like it or you don't."

Dorothy Draper

37
Have a hobby

Many people struggle to find time and energy for their hobbies and interests outside of work. However, pursuing your passions can have positive effects on your wellbeing, creativity, as well as productivity in other areas of your life. I hope that through this you will learn some ways to prioritise hobbies and interests outside of work and make them part of your routine.

The first thing to do is assess your values and goals. What do you enjoy doing? What makes you happy and fulfilled? What skills or knowledge do you want to develop or improve? Block out time in your calendar for them and stick to it. If possible, set a regular time and place for your hobby so that it becomes part of your routine and habit.

Do not overdo or neglect any aspect of your life, whether it is work, family, health, or leisure. Find a balance that works for you and that allows you to meet your obligations and needs. Also, diversify your hobbies and interests so that you can explore different facets of yourself and avoid boredom or burnout. Try new things, challenge yourself, and have fun.

Find people who share your hobbies and interests or who are willing to support you in pursuing them. Join online or offline communities, clubs, or groups that offer opportunities to interact, learn, and collaborate with others. Share your progress, achievements, and challenges with your friends, family, or social media followers. By connecting and sharing, you can enhance your social and emotional wellbeing, as well as gain feedback, inspiration, and encouragement.

Take time to review your hobbies and interests and how they have contributed to your growth, happiness, and satisfaction. Acknowledge your efforts, achievements, and improvements, as well as the challenges and obstacles you have overcome.

Express gratitude for the opportunities, resources, and people that have helped you along the way. By reflecting and appreciating, you can reinforce your positive attitude, self-esteem, and sense of purpose.

Recognise that your hobbies and interests may change over time, depending on your circumstances, preferences, and goals. Be flexible and open to new possibilities, and do not hesitate to try something different or let go of something that no longer serves you.

Also, be mindful of your limits and boundaries: do not force yourself to do something that you do not enjoy or that harms your wellbeing. By adapting and adjusting, you can maintain your interest, passion, and balance in your life.

Do you have a hobby?

What is your favourite hobby?

Do you take time out to work on your hobby regularly?

Is your hobby a pastime or is it something you would like to do full time?

"When diet is wrong, medicine is of no use.
When diet is correct, medicine is of no need."

Ayurvedic proverb

38

Eat for your body type

The elemental energies (air, water, fire, ether, and earth) influence everything from your physical shape and digestion to the way you process your thoughts and emotions.

Sometimes life, though, has a way of upsetting the balance in our body and this is where what you eat is vitally important. Ayurveda uses food as a way to balance your body when it is out of balance.

If your body is dominant with the vata dosha, then your body is made up mostly of air and ether which is usually light, cool, and dry in nature. People with a Vata constitution need to avoid dry cold food, especially vegetables. You can offset some of the coldness by adding a spicy oily dressing.

It is preferable to have warm, heavy, spicy, and oily foods with sour, salty, and sweet tastes. It is best to avoid cold drinks as they slow the digestion process down. Your vata will be out of balance if you have mild achiness, occasional constipation, or sleep or mood imbalances.

Because the pitta dosha is made up of fire and water and is sharp, oily, and hot, people with a dominant pitta dosha will benefit from cooling, heavy, dry foods with sweet, bitter, and astringent (green & black tea, beans, dried fruit apples, pears pomegranates) tastes. Avoid the salty, pungent (chillies, garlic, ginger & onion) and sour (citrus, vinegar, pickles & yoghurt) tastes as they will heat your system!

You will know if your pitta is out of balance because you will become irritable and impatient, and you may have occasional heartburn and acid reflux. You will be sensitive to heat and have skin rashes, acne, low blood sugar, and find it difficult to fall asleep.

People with a dominant kapha dosha in their body tend to benefit from adding heating spices to their diet, like pepper and ginger. Eat plenty of fresh vegetables, legumes, and fruit. The food needs to be lighter using bitter, astringent, and pungent foods. Avoid heavy, oily foods as well as those that are sweet, salty, and sour, and avoid eating large meals late at night.

You will know that your kapha is out of balance if you feel depressed, fatigued, lazy, apathetic, or you are gaining weight and suffering from coughs cold and congestion.

There is an art to maintaining balance by following a diet and a lifestyle best suited to your body type, like eating three meals a day at approximately the same time. Eat your biggest meal at lunchtime when your digestion is the strongest.

After reading this, do you have an inkling of your body type?

There is a link in the resources section where you can do the test.

Are there foods that you eat that maybe your body doesn't like?

Knowing your dosha will help you understand yourself and other people around you better.

"Never get so busy making a living that you forget to make a life."

Dolly Parton

39

Create a work-play balance

One of the most common regrets of people on their deathbed was that they spent too much time working and not enough time with the people they loved. A lot of people fall into the trap of working long hours, thinking that they can be more productive, but instead, they become stressed and maybe less productive than they would like to be. You can be as productive, if not more, by working 8 hours a day rather than 10 hours.

Overworking not only negatively affects you, but it can also affect your family. Workaholics and those who struggle to practise self-care find themselves at higher risk for burnout, fatigue, and stress-related health issues.

What does a work-play balance mean, and why is it so important? A work-play balance is when you have enough time to pursue both work and any personal interests that you love doing, whether that is spending time with your children or pursuing your own hobby.

People need rest as well as work, and they need variety so that their life is interesting – that can also positively impact their work life. You may find that creating the physical and mental space when you aren't thinking about work means ideas spontaneously drop into your mind, so it isn't like your play doesn't help your work.

It is critical that you know your values because you don't want to be engaging in an activity that doesn't bring you joy or isn't fun for you. Spend some time thinking about what is important to you in life and learning what your values are. It is very important that you take measures to find a work-play balance that works for you by setting clear boundaries, maybe by defining work hours that gives you time for relaxation as well as play.

Other things you could do is manage your time more efficiently by time blocking and checking how you spend your time. Maybe there are things that could be delegated to someone else, allowing you to have more time with your family or your hobbies.

Practising mindfulness also helps you to tune in to your feelings and your body, and it makes you more aware of when something isn't congruent with your goals, for instance. Managing your stress levels is important for your health, not only now, but in your future as well, since stress leads to many health issues like digestive problems, inability to sleep, and possibly high blood pressure leading to a heart attack or stroke.

I know that for workaholics this is probably something you will have to work on, but it will be worth it. Imagine how productive you will be when you are rested and your cup is full!

Are you one of the lucky ones that has a great work-play balance?

Are you too exhausted when you get home from work to do anything?

What could be one thing you do to correct your work-play balance?

Start to make changes this week!

"A man is getting old when he walks around a puddle instead of through it."

R C Ferguson

40

Let your inner child play

Children as they are growing up are usually happy. They are curious little beings and see the magic, wonder, and amazement in everything that is all around them. They are so creative and don't worry about what others think.

So why don't they all grow up to be adults with curiosity still in them, the joy for life, the learning and the appreciation for all that is around them? It is almost like at some point they are told that they cannot associate with that child from now on – only be an adult.

However, there are unfortunate events that some children experience that take them away from their child nature. Maybe they have to take on an adult role as I did, after my father passed away and I cooked for my family. Others have been traumatised, or they were looking after a parent, or had a broken family. These experiences can cause children to become adults much too early and they lose touch with their inner child far too soon.

As adults, we are generally uncomfortable expressing ourselves. We tend to channel all our thoughts and emotions and bottle it up to become the adult person we think we should be. In this process you lose what you originally were as a child and so – poof! – we lose touch with the child inside.

Others lose their inner child by surrendering to the pressures of society. Once you become an adult, then you are expected to act like an adult. Heaven help us if we do express our inner child and people should laugh at us or think we are childish!

Though I know how to do the adulting thing when it is needed, I also can transform into the child-like Mama Rae at other times. It makes life interesting and humorous as well as light hearted, and I think that is vital, especially in these busy and serious times we live in.

Though you might not feel connected to your inner child, they're always there. I believe keeping in touch with your inner child has many benefits. It keeps you feeling young; it stops you from getting too serious about not only yourself but your life as well; it allows you to have a light hearted attitude towards many aspects of life. Appreciation of the little things you have in your life is the same as being grateful.

Let go of judgment and release your fear of what other people think and be a kid again. Feel the pleasure in all the little things, the sunsets, the blooming flowers, random smiles from strangers.

When was the last time you sat and watched the sun rise or set?

When was the last time you felt as free as a child?

Have you recently danced because you felt full of joy?

When was the last time you walked through a puddle?

"*All disease begins in the gut.*"

Hippocrates

41
The fire of life

Most of us don't realise how much poor digestive health affects our body. It can lead to autoimmune disease, allergies, chronic fatigue, mood disorders, and dementia among others. It is important, therefore, to have a proper working gut for us to have good health.

Simplified, the digestive process extracts the energy you need to live and eliminates what is left behind. The entire process can take between 10 and 73 hours and depends on what you have eaten as well as the portion size. Carbohydrates will take around two or three hours, while animal protein and fish can take up to two days to fully digest.

The process of digestion, including absorption and assimilation, begins in the mouth. Enzymes in the saliva soften what we eat. Amylase breaks down complex carbohydrates into sugars and lipase breaks down fats.

The longer you chew food, the closer it will get to a paste-like substance which makes it easier for the stomach to break it down further. Food that hasn't been chewed for long enough won't necessarily be fully digested, and so you won't get all the nutrients in the food.

Once the paste in the stomach is turned acidic by hydrochloric acid for further digestion by pepsin and gastrin, the stomach's strong muscles work like a blender to transform the food so it is usable by our body. It then enters the small intestines where this acid is neutralised, which allows bile and pancreatic juices to further digest it and pass it, finally, along to the large intestine for the last stage of digestion and the elimination of wastes.

There are some 500 species of bacteria in our gut helping to digest the food, regulate hormones, produce vitamins, and eliminate toxins. If you happen to have too many bad bugs like yeasts and parasites and not enough of the good bacteria, then that is most likely where you will start to have health problems.

Sluggish digestion will lower your immunity, and you could become more susceptible to cough, colds, and other diseases going around.

So, it is vitally important to look after your digestive fire and digestive processes, and it's best not to eat when you are angry, upset, or sad – having regular eating times helps too.

Are you hungry when you eat?

Do you have acid reflux after eating?

Do you have bloating after you have eaten?

Do you have a large drink with your meal?

"*If you realised how powerful your thoughts are, you would never think a negative thought.*"

Peace Pilgrim

42

Be mindful of your self-talk

elf-talk is your inner voice, the messages you send to yourself throughout each day. For some of us, that voice can be decidedly negative. Negative self-talk is when your inner voice behaves exclusively like a critic. It is pessimistic and focuses on the bad, erodes your confidence, and stops you from reaching your potential. It can make you feel like you are going to fail before you even start.

This inner voice combines our conscious thoughts with inbuilt beliefs and biases. As adults we have internalised lessons from childhood and our families that have led us to believe that maybe we aren't good enough or that we are always doing things wrong.

So, let me ask you this: are you the sort of person who automatically sees the problem in any situation or the solution? Many of us automatically think in a negative way. Initially, we see how something will impede our path or how a situation will turn out badly rather than having a neutral or balanced outlook. Let me put it another way: think of yourself as a magnet. If your core is negativity, you are going to radiate that negative magnetic field into the world.

You may engage in negative self-talk just some of the time, or it might be all-consuming. Either way, negative self-talk tears us down, leads us to unfounded and unnecessary feelings of shame, which can impact our relationships.

Thinking of taxes causes our blood pressure to rise, so does being late for a meeting or contemplating how to pay for a home improvement that's just out of our budget. In none of these instances does our fight or flight response serve a purpose. All it does is get us agitated and makes our heart beat faster. It prepares us to run, but to where and to what end?

Right now, there are people everywhere who feel anxious, ready to run from modern day predators that seem scary, but in reality, don't amount to much. Our misplaced anxiety can seem silly at times (especially when after frantically searching for 15 minutes the keys were in the same place you left them), but it is still a serious problem that can cost money and can cost lives.

Let go of the stories you've been telling yourself. Let go of the victim role you are playing. Observe your thoughts from a distance and let them go, instead of attaching emotions to them. Change your environment. Be mindful of who you listen to, what you eat, and who you are spending time with.

Raise your energy to live a more peaceful, loving life, and at the same time, you will help those around you do the same.

Be mindful of your self-talk

Do you have a repetitive theme in your self-talk?

Are you aware of what your self-talk is?

Are you able to still your mind?

Can you instantly list things that you think will be a problem?

"The New Age? It's just the old age stuck in a microwave oven for fifteen seconds."

James Randi

43

Minimise the microwave

Not long after I bought my first microwave, I read an article which suggested that waves changed the molecular structure of food cooked in a microwave, at which point I stopped using it. Further research suggests that this isn't the case. I find it just as easy to reheat food on the stovetop. To get the best out of your microwave, I feel there are some dos and don'ts that need to be taken into consideration.

Phthalates are one of the most common ingredients used to make plastic more flexible. They are in takeaway containers, plastic wrap, plastic water bottles, toys, body lotions, and containers. They are everywhere, but unfortunately, phthalates have also been found to disrupt our hormones as well as our metabolism.

In children, they can increase blood pressure and insulin resistance, increasing the risk of diabetes. Bisphenol is also used in plastic products, which may also be a hormone disrupter, although at this point how much damage it causes is not yet clear.

Most of us would have an array of plastic containers in our cupboards and drawers which are used for heating food in the microwave. Though it's important to remember that when heating food in a plastic container, exposure also can happen with plastic that doesn't touch the food, such as a lid.

Water rises as steam from the food, and then condenses on the underside of the lid, and the chemicals from the lid then fall into your food. If you use plastic wrap, then make sure it doesn't touch the food. You could use absorbent paper towel in place of the plastic wrap.

The best ways to minimise risk are to use other microwave-safe materials like plastic containers made for that purpose, glass containers, and ceramic containers.

If you do use plastic containers, avoid any that are losing their shape since old and damaged containers are more likely to leach chemicals. To check your container, look for the recycling symbol on the base of the container. If you see the letters "V" or "PVC" with the number 3, then it contains phthalates.

It's important to note that reheating food also has its risks. Food should be heated to 82°C throughout to kill any harmful bacteria, so you do need to stir the food during heating. Bacteria can grow each time food cools down, so it is best not to reheat your meal more than once.

Is your food hot all the way through when you eat it?

What do you reheat your food in?

Do you reheat food a second time?

Do you use a microwave?

"Talk to yourself like you would to someone you love."

Brené Brown

44

Be kind to yourself

I think most of us find it easier to be kind to others rather than to ourselves. It is so ingrained in us that we do something for someone else we don't even think about it. It is like we haven't trained our mind to think about ourselves like that. Yet being kind to ourselves helps our mental health and wellbeing.

Showing kindness to ourselves is helpful, especially when things don't go the way we would like or expect them to. Our inner voice would have more than likely been critical and see it the totally opposite way from how a friend would.

So having that encouraging inner voice tell us it is OK that we failed or made a mistake – as you would say to a friend – would bolster our self-confidence immensely.

Showing self-compassion can also help us cope with anxiety and stress and helps us feel more satisfied with life. The next time you do something kind for a friend, think about doing something for yourself. Spend some time each day speaking kindly to yourself, even if it is only for five minutes.

Try to become conscious and more aware of when you are voicing negative things to yourself. Try saying them out loud when they are more likely to make an impact. They can also make you more resilient when things go awry in the future.

Make time each day to focus on how you are feeling. Write it in a journal. This will help you recognise faster when your inner voice is being critical.

Some other things you could do are:

- **Creating healthy routines** that are great self-care, like having a healthy breakfast, going for a walk, and spending time on your hobbies.

- Take time out each day for **meditation or mindfulness** to help you become more present in the here and now rather than worrying about the past or the future.

- **Spend time in nature,** whether it is at the beach, by the river, or in a park. Nature has a way of calming us and bringing us back to ourselves, making you take notice of what is happening around you. Leave your phone at home.

- If you have a challenging day at work, then **think about what you are doing.** If you reach for the alcohol or be tempted to eat unhealthy food, take a walk and then see how you feel afterwards.

Are you too stressed to think about yourself?

Do you remember the last thing you thought about yourself was?

What ways are you kind to yourself?

When was the last time you spent time working on your hobby?

"Never give up on a dream just because of the time it will take to accomplish it. The time will pass anyway."

Earl Nightingale

45
Write a bucket list

A bucket list is a list of things one would like to either experience or achieve before you pass into the next life. These words can remind us of our own mortality and death is not something we readily talk about, much less think about.

But it is wise to remember that time is limited as we age but is also one of the best gifts we are given. It is a nudge for us to know what we want to achieve and what is most important to us before it is too late, and we then regret not getting them done.

It isn't necessarily a fixed list, as it may change as you grow older and your needs and wishes change. Things that may seem impossible can become attainable accomplishments by having them on the list as you become used to seeing them. You can change your thinking from I could never do that to how can I do it.

The great thing about having a bucket list is that it keeps you in touch with your dreams and what is important to you. Maybe you have lived your life to now doing what you felt was expected of you, perhaps not even aware of what you would love to do.

Having the list is a great motivation to achieve things in our lives because it forces us to look at our life and decide if that is what we want it to be moving forward.

If there is a life you would rather be living, then your list can provide you with the motivation to do that. Some of the things you have on your list might seem impossible, but don't focus on the 'how' just keep focusing on it being on your list, until it feels comfortable.

Then you will have conviction that you will get it done. It will give you energy and give meaning behind the effort to work that extra hour and create excitement deep in your soul that you haven't had.

Writing your bucket list down will have more of an impact and you are more likely to make it happen than if you just have it in your mind. It will give you a sense of direction and will less likely be distracted by unimportant things. Keeping your focus on your goals will help you live the rich and full life you all deserve. Accomplishment gives you a feeling of pride, which in turn builds self-esteem and increases life satisfaction.

If you don't have a list, start one. They don't have to be huge ones like climb Mount Everest or ride a bike around the world, but it could be if that's what floats your boat! Maybe you have been wanting to grow your own vegetables or travel around Australia or even just write a book. No matter what is on your list, make sure it is what you want to do and not what somebody else says you should do. Okay, now start writing!

Do you have a bucket list?

What is one thing on your bucket list you would love to do?

Is there anything on your list that doesn't seem possible?

What will be your first priority?

"If you think more about those around you, then you find you worry less about yourself."

Unknown

46
Keep the magic alive

The early stages in our relationships are usually fun and filled with surprises, when there is so much to learn and discover about each other.

Getting to know each other strengthens the bond between you; however, over time, when life becomes busy and your attention is taken away from your relationship, then the freshness and joy can fade and become predictable. Every time I go shopping, I see men following their wives, pushing the trolley looking like they would rather be anywhere else but in the supermarket.

A connection with a partner does not evolve without effort from both people in the relationship, as I found out in my last relationship. I wanted to grow and become a better version of myself, so I started doing courses to help me do that.

My husband, on the other hand, was content to be the same person, doing the same thing day in and day out. So, it probably was no surprise that the relationship fizzled out because it does take the both of you to grow.

What can you do to help keep the magic in your relationship? I think that it is worth remembering that you were both madly in love in the beginning, so underneath the boring, mundane monotony, the love is probably still there; it just needs to be rekindled and fed.

The key to adding excitement into your relationship is continually pursuing new experiences together while also finding new ways to demonstrate that you value each other. Look for experiences that will reinvigorate your appreciation for each other. Go on regular dates, especially to do things you haven't done before or explore new places you don't know. Take time to go away for the weekend to places you haven't been before so you can create new memories.

Do you know their love language? You can tailor your gifts to them using their love language. If they show their love through touch, then they would probably appreciate a massage or a shoulder rub, especially after a busy day at the office. Check to see if you are really listening to your partner and that he/she feels understood rather than thinking about your own problems or issues while they are speaking to you.

These are the things that keep us awake and growing as individuals, and they keep our relationships alive, fun, and flourishing. If you want the quality of your relationship to be extraordinary and long-lasting, then you need to continually put in your time and effort to ensure that it stays that way.

When was the last time you laughed and had fun together
with your partner?

When did you last do something spontaneous?

When did you last go somewhere you haven't been before?

When did you last surprise your partner?

"Sleep is the interest we have to pay on the capital, which is called in at death, and the higher the rate of interest the more regularly it is paid, the further the date of redemption is postponed."

Arthur Schopenhauer

47

Sleep is important

My sleep became nothing short of disastrous when I was running my coffee shop. I opened the café at 6:30am and closed it at 6:30pm, then I went shopping for what was needed for the next day. By the time I got home, it was 8:00pm and I was so dog-tired that I would fall asleep in a chair and wake up around midnight. Unfortunately, I couldn't fall asleep again when I went to bed, so having four hours a night was the pattern of my sleep for several years.

Sleep plays a vital role in good health and wellbeing all through your life, from childhood to old age. The way you feel while you are awake depends for the most part on what happens while you are sleeping. During sleep, your body is working to support healthy brain function and to maintain your physical health. Teens and small children, especially, need good sleep in order to support their growth and development.

Lack of sleep can lead to long-term chronic health problems. These include decreased physical activity with no desire to exercise together with higher levels of the hormones regulating your hunger, making you more likely to eat not only more food but more fatty and sweet foods.

Not having enough sleep increases the risk of having poor mental health as well as an inability to focus on tasks and think clearly. Good sleep is just as important in improving our health as having a healthy diet and exercise.

It is also important to look at your bedroom. Is there much light coming in at night? I didn't realise how important it was to have a blacked-out room to sleep in until I was staying with my daughter, Cassie in Auckland. No light at all came into the room once the curtains were closed. I had the best sleep ever, waking refreshed every morning. It wasn't just my body; it was my mind that benefited immensely from the deep sleep I was having. It felt so much more alert.

Of course, it makes sense that one would sleep deeper in a darkened room than one with light. Our unconscious mind would need to be on alert for any possible danger meaning that your sleep wouldn't be as deep.

While there is no right or wrong number of hours each person needs, it is probably more important that you go to sleep at the same time each night. Limit your use of television, computer screens, and your phones at night, all of which can make it harder to fall asleep.

OK, time for bed – good night!

How many hours did you sleep last night?

How did you feel when you woke up?

If you are waking up at the same time during the night, what time is it?

What time do you go to sleep?

"Healthy does NOT mean starving yourself EVER. Healthy means eating the right food in the right amount."

Karen Salmansohn

48
Eat well on a budget

I found out how inexpensive eating healthy could be when I was in New Zealand with my daughter, Cassie, during Covid in 2020. When I arrived, I didn't realise that I could only use one of my bank cards, which, at the time, had only $50 on it.

I bought the food I needed and was pleasantly surprised to find that I had money left over at the end of the week. So, I would like to share with you some of the things I do that allows me to eat healthy and cheaply.

The number one thing is that I never ever go shopping when I am hungry. It is too tempting to buy snacks that are not only expensive but aren't necessarily nutritious. Plus, they won't sustain you for as long as any healthy meal will. Those foods are generally at head height on the supermarket shelves for a reason, knowing you will buy them on an impulse.

Before you go shopping, check your pantry and fridge to see what is in there that could be used. There may be food that is about to expire or hidden from sight, but it could be included in your next meal, so you do not waste it.

Plan out some meals for a few days or for the week so that you will have a shopping list of things you know you are going to use. If you buy vegetables for five days ahead, they may go to waste if your plans change or, say, you decide to go out for dinner with friends one night. It is much more practical to buy vegetables for the next two or three days only.

Use leftovers on toast for breakfast the next morning or use them for lunches or in other recipes like stews, stir-fries, salads and burritos. Try replacing meat in more meals with eggs, beans, seeds, vegetables, and whole grains instead – or use cheaper cuts of meat. Wholefoods are less expensive than the processed ones and on top of that, they are more nutritious!

Many processed foods often contain lots of salt and sugar, along with artificial flavours and preservatives which are less healthy.

To lower the cost of your food, you could buy foods in bulk, like beans, quinoa, and millet, which is usually cheaper. Buy the generic brand that supermarkets have or stock up on staples when they are on special.

Just by eliminating any processed food, you should find that your grocery shop will be less expensive and healthier.

You can buy cans of chickpeas, black beans, cannellini beans or red kidney beans that with the addition of some spices and vegetables can make a delicious and nutritious meal up quickly and you don't have to be a cordon bleu chef to be able do it.

Do you go shopping with a list of what you need?

How much food do you throw out each week?

How much of your food is processed food?

Do you need to learn how to cook?

"The nontoxic life is not expensive, it's priceless."

Unknown

49

Use non-toxic cleaners

Cleaning is in an essential and regular part of all our lives. But I ask you this question: how often do you read the labels on the cleaning products you buy? While there are many benefits to keeping our living spaces clean, there are some products that can be a health risk. Cleaning products contain many chemicals that are toxic and can affect your body when you use them.

The toxins enter your body when you inhale the fumes and you also absorb the chemicals through your skin, especially through your hands. The problem is made worse because your hands are often wet when you are doing the cleaning, which damages the skin's protective barrier, allowing the chemicals to be absorbed more easily.

There are several short-term effects as well, including skin irritations and rashes, worsening of asthma conditions, and shortness of breath, which can be caused by chlorine bleach in cleaners.

So, what are the ones you need to be aware of?

Sodium hydroxide, ammonium hydroxide, and chlorine bleach are often found in oven and drain cleaners. These are corrosive and irritating chemicals which can cause serious skin burns, eye damage, and breathing problems.

Carpet and upholstery cleaners contain naphthalene, perchloroethylene, and ammonium hydroxide, which can release fumes that can cause short-term effects like nausea and dizziness. If you are using these cleaners, then make sure you have plenty of fresh air in the room.

Most antibacterial cleaners, apart from containing surfactants, also have a pesticide, typically either phenolic chemicals or quaternary ammonium, both of which can burn your skin and throat and irritate your eyes.

Oven cleaners can emit toxic fumes and cause chemical burns if exposed to your skin. They can become highly dangerous if not cleaned thoroughly before turning on your oven to cook. Your non-stick frying pans can become toxic if they get scratched, so always use wooden spoons when cooking with them.

Even laundry detergents can be harmful. Any detergent with "cationic" or "non-ionic" ingredients can cause skin irritations and eye damage.

For thirty years I have used vinegar to clean the toilet and the wooden floors, wet newspaper to clean the windows; I make an enzyme cleaner for general cleaning and a shower cleaner with borax and vinegar. Ovens can be cleaned using vinegar, baking soda, and aluminium foil.

I also make my own laundry detergent and hand wash. They might not work for you, but you could try experimenting with them.

Have you read the list of ingredients on your cleaners?

Do you notice any symptoms after you use them?

Do you need all the cleaners you have in your cupboard?

Would you like to change any of them?

"*You are not your mistakes; they are what you did, not who you are.*"

Lisa Lieberman-Wang

50

You are not your mistakes

I am certain that none of you would be able to write a list of every mistake you have ever made, much less the ones you made in the past month – that is if you did make any!

Many of the things that we have done and consider to be mistakes probably won't be seen in the years to come the same way as it felt when they happened. You will have forgotten about them or maybe even seen the blessings in them. Really, it may not even take one or two months to forget about most of them.

It is so easy to label our actions as mistakes in our mind especially when we have 60,000 thoughts a day. So, why do we get so attached to making a mistake?

Unfortunately, we all have a inner critic who is so fast at reminding us of what we believe about ourselves, that we are lazy, stupid, dumb, that we choose to believe that is why we made the mistake, rather than change our mindset to have a different belief about the mistake.

Maybe it is because we try to get things right; we try to be a perfectionist to make ourselves feel good enough. However, labels aren't necessarily useful, especially because the negative ones limit us, and they certainly don't help us feel good about ourselves.

I think most of us see our mistakes and feel we have failed in some way. But consider this, if we didn't make mistakes, how would we learn to do something the right way or get the desired outcome we are looking for? Imagine if scientists stopped their experiment because they made a mistake or if a chef never tried a recipe a second time just because they made a mistake on the first attempt?

We all have our own expectations for ourselves in different areas of our lives, and I think when we fail or make a mistake, it impacts how we define ourselves. We tell ourselves that we are "useless" or "not good enough". It is pointless to define ourselves by something outside of us because it is out of our control anyway. The truth is you are not your mistakes.

One way to look at mistakes is rather than seeing them as mistakes, see them as miss-takes, giving you the opportunity to try again and get it right – or just look at them as furthering your education.

Remember that your value is intrinsic as well as unconditional, so no matter what miss-takes you make you are still you, in all your magnificence. So, love yourself, accept yourself, and value yourself for who you are and let your mistakes become lessons you can learn from instead.

How many of your mistakes do you remember?

What do you tell yourself when you make a mistake?

How do you feel after you realise you made a mistake?

What do you learn from making a mistake?

"Smoking may offer temporary relief, but quitting will grant you a lifetime of freedom and vitality."

Unknown

51

No smoking

For those of you who know me, it might be a shock to you that I smoked for twenty years! It might be an even bigger shock to you after you read this story:

As a trainee nurse, I witnessed my first autopsy. The doctor cut out the woman's liver, which was twice the normal size and covered with lumps, and he said, "This is what happens when you drink." Next, he showed me her lungs and squeezed them. A smelly black liquid oozed out and he said, "This is what happens when you smoke."

I was so distressed by this that afterwards I went and bought my first packet of cigarettes!

Over the next twenty years, I tried everything from acupuncture to hypnosis to help me stop. In the end, it was a severe case of tonsilitis which made the decision easy. I couldn't smoke, eat, drink, or talk, and so I decided that this was sent to me by a higher power. I have been a non-smoker for almost 40 years, and thankfully my body has fully recovered.

I totally understand why you would want to smoke. I don't want to come across as a scaremonger, but I also don't want to sugarcoat it: if you are a smoker, I want you to know what your future may hold for you.

It is known that smokers lose bone density at a faster rate, leaving you open to breaking a bone or hip. Smoking puts you at higher risk of developing type 2 diabetes in addition to other increased risks of complications due to poor circulation, including amputation of a limb.

For women who smoke, there can be several issues. Smoking can affect your ability to conceive because it reduces your fertility. If you have an ectopic pregnancy, where the egg implants outside the uterus, this puts your life at risk. Orofacial clefts are caused when a baby's lips or mouth don't develop as they should, and these occur more often in a woman who smokes.

So now you want to quit smoking? That's great news! Make a difference by changing the way you do things and your environment. Move your desk to a different place. Redecorate your space, change your dinner time, even change your drink, and buy yourself a stress ball to hold in your smoking hand.

The more options you give yourself, the easier it will be to help your brain to break the link between what you are doing and cigarettes. Each time you resist the urge to have a cigarette, you are one step closer to being a non-smoker.

Good luck!

Have you tried to give up smoking?

Are you concerned about your health?

Do you have lung problems?

Do you find yourself coughing a lot?

"*Reduce inflammation to treat the root of many issues. If your gut isn't working right, it can cause so many other issues.*"

Jay Woodman

52

Eat anti-inflammatory foods

Inflammation is part of the body's defence mechanism. It signals for the immune system to fight off infection and heal injuries. There are two types of inflammation: acute and chronic. Acute inflammation occurs when you have cut yourself, you have a fever, you've twisted your ankle, or you have diarrhoea after eating something bad. Acute inflammation is part of the healing process.

Chronic inflammation, on the other hand, results from slow, long-term inflammation over many months and even years. It can damage healthy cells, tissues, and even organs. It is the key factor that causes almost all chronic degenerative diseases.

Some symptoms of chronic inflammation are anxiety, insomnia, depression, frequent infections, gastrointestinal problems like diarrhoea, chronic tiredness, and constipation, as well as body pain and weight loss or gain. Unfortunately, chronic inflammation is happening in your body without you realising it.

A few risk factors that are underlying chronic inflammation include irregular sleep patterns, stress, smoking, obesity, age, and diet. Of these, it is diet that I want to talk to you about. The main inflammatory foods are processed foods, damaged trans-fats, simple sugars, refined carbohydrates, hydrogenated oils, and high glycaemic foods.

Although chronic inflammation progresses silently, it is the cause of most chronic diseases and presents a major threat to the health and longevity of individuals. Inflammation is considered a major contributor to several diseases including cardiovascular diseases, diabetes, arthritis, and other joint diseases, together with lung diseases.

Now let's get to the nitty gritty of this subject – food. Firstly, the main task for you is to limit the intake of inflammation-producing foods like soft drinks, refined carbohydrates, and anything which has fructose or corn syrup on the label – also, processed foods, like lunch meats, pies, cakes, French fries and fried chicken. If you avoid these foods, you will be off to a good start.

The next thing would be to reduce the number of foods you consume that contain trans fats, like processed seed and vegetable oils. Replace them with coconut oil, olive oil, or avocado oil. All these oils have a higher smoking point, which is the temperature at which oils burn.

Foods to include in your diet would be those that are high in antioxidants and other anti-inflammatory compounds, like blueberries, cauliflower, broccoli, apples, nuts, and fish oil – also mung beans and turmeric, which contains curcumin.

Many of these foods will give you the micronutrients to help reduce inflammation that might otherwise increase the risk of various chronic diseases.

Do you eat a lot of inflammatory foods?

How often do you eat anti-inflammatory foods?

Do you notice any inflammation in your sinuses after eating
those foods?

Do you suffer from bloating after eating?

"Not knowing when the dawn will come, I open every door."

Emily Dickinson

53

Say yes to life

Many of us automatically think in a negative way. With any suggestion, people commonly see what won't work or why it is wrong or bad, and so they won't try anything new or different because they initially see the results as negative. Or there are people whose lives become so humdrum and boring that they settle into a routine of seriousness and don't see the magic around them anymore.

I know that if you were to think of yourself as a magnet and you think negatively, then that is the energy you will put out into the world... but it doesn't have to be that way!

Whether your energy came from a learned way life that you have inherited from a parent, or it happened organically through your life events (and your reaction to those), everyone has the choice to change their attitude. You just need to be aware of what your life is turning into and decide that isn't the life you want to lead.

So rather than working yourself to death, try spending some valuable time doing things that are important to you. Start saying yes to things you would have said no to previously and see what happens; see how it changes you and your life.

It doesn't have to be a perfect fit at first. Get yourself out there and meet new people. Do things you haven't tried but always wanted to, without automatically seeing the downfall or negative aspect of it. Experience new adventures and take new opportunities to test yourself. You will find that at work you will be more productive and maybe even enjoy it more.

You may find that you enjoy saying yes without even thinking negatively about it. That will be a marker of how far you have come! It is possible you will find that thinking positively rather than negatively becomes the norm for you.

Try meditating so you can become more aware of your thoughts. This practice will make it easier to monitor your negative thoughts and then change them before you speak. This will also help you say yes to more things rather than saying no.

You could start seeing the good in bad situations, rather than just seeing the negative side. Are you reading my mind? Of course, I am also going to say look at the food you are eating, because after all, a healthy body goes a long way to creating a healthy mind.

Stop trying to control everything and just let life happen when you say YES to life.

Are you a person who says "No" to opportunities?

Is your life an incredibly busy one?

Do you find yourself saying "No" to things and experiences you would love?

What is the worst thing that could happen if you did say "Yes"?

"Strive not to be a success, but rather to be of value."

Albert Einstein

54
Value yourself for what you know

When my daughter Emily said to me that I should write this book and that I ought to write down all the things I do that allow me to be vital and alive, I was stunned when I got to 75! I honestly expected maybe reaching 35 to 40 different things.

Yet there they were for all to see. It was at this point that I felt compelled to acknowledge that I had learned a thing or three over the years. It is something that we don't usually think about, much less acknowledge.

However, in going through the process of putting in all the knowledge and wisdom I had gained from my experiences over the years into perspective, I had to recognise that I had learned a lot. I feel that I have a lot to be grateful for having had the life I have experienced. At the same time, I know I have a lot to pass on to those of you who are ready and want it.

Positive thoughts about ourselves create neural connections that are strengthened every time you think about them. The stronger the connections, the more it shapes what you believe to be true about what you can or cannot learn. Your mindset influences not only your thoughts and emotions but also your results.

By acknowledging and celebrating yourself more often, you physically alter your brain to notice more evidence of your capabilities and successes. You can programme yourself to believe that you can learn anything and that you are capable of creating positive changes in your life as a result.

As you strengthen those belief systems, you can experience even more confidence and resilience. So I invite you to pause for a brief moment now to appreciate one thing that you may have learned this week.

Many of us tend to under-appreciate the "minor" things we learn every day because we more easily remember more expansive things, such as those times when we made a mistake or "failed" at something, and we tend to focus on what we learned from those experiences.

The seemingly small things we learn can have an impact as big as anything we consider to have been a huge learning.

In the next few days list out the topics you know about and the add the random things you have learned that made an impact on you.

Are there small things you've learned that you apply to your life?

Have you listed the different subjects you have learned about?

What about things you know?

Have you ever taken the time to appreciate how much you know?

"A friend is someone who knows the song in your heart and can sing it back to you when you have forgotten the words."

Shania Twain

55
Have friends that bring you joy

Humans have been wired to have social interactions from the beginning. Our social connections are a survival mechanism. Our friends provide us with feelings of being safe, loved, and supported. Unfortunately, in our modern times we are more disconnected than ever before, separated from our family and friends.

It is interesting to note that social isolation and loneliness are associated with having a weaker immune system, and this is true across all generations. Without social connections and friends, our brain goes into flight or fight mode and that can lead to anxiety and stress. It isn't so important that you have a lot of friends, but the quality of the relationship is what is more important.

True friends can have a major effect on your health and wellbeing. They are beside you celebrating the good times just as they are in your corner supporting you when you need them. Adults with strong social connections generally have less significant health problems like depression and high blood pressure.

For older people, friends prevent them from feeling isolated and alone. Developing friendships can take effort, but the benefits are well worth it. Those who have meaningful relationships with friends tend to live longer. Having friends gives us a sense of belonging, which is important for everyone's sense of wellbeing.

Friends tend to keep us on our toes, reminding us of our strengths, boosting our self-confidence and self-worth, which helps increase our sense of purpose and belonging. They are also there when we are coping with any of life's trauma, no matter whether it is an illness, a job loss, or a separation; they are there giving us positive encouragement.

They are there looking out for you and keeping you accountable if you are drinking too much, working too many hours, or not exercising. Great friends encourage you to have healthy habits. The emotional support from friends is invaluable, especially when you are grieving a loved one. Good friends also inspire us when things are tough.

They keep us grounded and help us remember our values, our strengths, and what our purpose in life is, not to mention teach us new things and give us a different perspective. They encourage us to become better versions of ourselves. Friends are kind, fun, compassionate, accept us for who we are, value our time, and respect our boundaries. They are true friends.

Do your friends bring you joy?

Do your friends value and appreciate you?

Is it time to re-evaluate the friends in your circle?

Is it time to let some go?

"What we've learned is that if you can make the right decision in the supermarket aisle, it's a heck of a lot easier to make a good decision when you reach in your cupboard when you're craving a snack at eight o'clock at night."

Tom Rath

56

Snack well

Ayurveda considers that snacking between meals weakens your digestive fire. If the snack is still in your stomach when you begin to eat your next meal, the gut must finish dealing with the snack before it can start digesting your main meal. The undigested food encourages fermentation, excess gas and bloating, and then the growth of bacteria results in a buildup of toxins.

The time between eating will vary from person to person. Two people can eat the same meal and one can be hungry two hours after and the other can be satisfied for three or four hours. While you shouldn't ignore hunger, you could check if it is real hunger and not thirst, boredom, or an emotional response by having a drink of water and check after 15 to 20 minutes to see if you are still hungry.

An individual's need for food varies, with some people needing to eat more often. For example, a person with a Pitta dosha can digest food faster and needs to eat more frequently than someone with a Vata or Kapha dosha. However, continual snacking means that there isn't enough time between meals for the food to be completely digested.

People generally will reach for either sweet or salty snacks, neither of which is good from a health aspect and can lead to mindless eating and overconsumption, straining the digestive system, causing imbalances and the formation of digestive toxins. The important thing is that you choose nourishing and easily digested foods as snacks.

The snack food industry is a bazillion dollar industry which mostly portrays the products as healthy, but they are heavily laced with additives. They are also strategically marketed to lure you into thinking that it the product is healthy.

When my older two children were at primary school, I started buying Tiny Teddies to add to their lunch box. They liked the chocolate ones and, as it turned out, I did too! One day, I thought I should try one. I had one and another and another. It got to the point where not even a week later I couldn't stop at four or five – I found I had eaten the entire packet. They were so addictive! That was the last packet I bought.

Dry foods are dehydrating at worst and aggravate your nervous system because of the extra air in the gut, so drink plenty of water. The best snacks have plenty of protein, healthy fats, and fibre.

Do you find yourself mindlessly snacking?

What do you snack on?

How healthy are your snacks?

Do you eat them because you are bored?

"Your diet is a bank account. Good food choices are investments."

Bethany Frankel

57

Substitution not deprivation

Eating well doesn't mean never enjoying your food. Gluten bread for breakfast used to make me feel sleepy later in the morning, so I decided I needed to replace it with something else. It was the same when I chose not to have dairy.

My main concerns at the time were what do I replace them with, and will I enjoy their taste? So now, 30 years later, I can tell you that I would never go back. The replacements are so much more sustaining, and the taste is way better than I ever thought it would be.

If you do want to cut out some foods from your diet, then I suggest you try replacing them with some healthier options and notice the difference in your physical, mental, and cognitive health.

Have a go at trying some of these food and drink replacements.

Replace parmesan cheese with nutritional yeast and I doubt you will notice the difference. I make a sauce of almonds, water, nutritional yeast, and Herbamare salt, which I add to lasagnes and other pasta dishes.

If it is difficult to change to a non-wheat bread, then try a sour dough bread which is easier to digest; it is richer in nutrients and it is also less likely to spike your blood sugar, because the fermentation process mostly breaks down the gluten.

Instead of a soft drink, try mixing sparkling water with an unsweetened fruit juice.

There are now plenty of vegan cheese options which taste so delicious.

Instead of butter or canola oil, you can use olive oil, ghee, or avocado oil.

Lower your sugar intake by using mustard in place of the sugar laden sauces.

Replace the wheat varieties of pastas with buckwheat, pea, or vegetable varieties. If you are making lasagne, you can use zucchini or eggplant, instead of the wheat lasagne sheets.

If you like chips/crisps, try making your own vegetable chips. They are easy to do and just as tasty if you add some herbs, a healthy oil, and garlic to thinly sliced vegetables.

When using oil to heat foods, try olive, coconut, or avocado oil which, when heated, don't burn at high temperatures like an unrefined oil.

Some of these may take time getting used to, but I am certain in the long run you will be pleased that you did. And take it slowly; you don't have to try to change everything at once. Change one thing at a time to see if you like them.

What unhealthy food would you like to change out first?

Are you aware of how you feel after eating these foods?

Does eating gluten make you feel tired?

Do you want to lower your sugar intake?

"Connecting with your spirit guide is like having a compass that never fails."

Unknown

58

We are not here alone

It was around 20 years after my dad had passed that I realised he had never really been missing. There was always a man in my life who had taken the place of my dad. First, it was my oldest brother; then in high school, it was my physics teacher who took me under his wing, listening to me and giving me advice.

After I left school, it would be my next-door neighbour or the man in the shop where I used to buy my jewellery. In essence, although my dad wasn't with me physically, he had never left me – energetically anyway. I came to realise from these relationships that we aren't here alone.

Once I realised that my dad wasn't missing from my life, I began talking with him, asking him questions, and letting him know how I was going. It doesn't matter if it is a loved one or God or the universe, knowing that there is a presence always there supporting you gives you an unfaltering faith and strength, whether you can 'see' them or not. That kept me feeling supported and moving forward, but things changed with Covid.

There was isolation during Covid times and people had to keep their distance from you when out shopping. People wouldn't look at you let alone speak to you, which I accepted like all of us, but unconsciously, I felt isolated. At the same time, I experienced a lot of grief and loss with loved ones passing and some leaving for other parts of the world.

All of this took its toll on my mental health, although at the time I didn't realise it. I just thought that I had, for some reason, lost my enthusiasm for life, and my inspiration and motivation had left me. I somehow lost contact with my father's spirit. Somewhere during the past two years I felt the problem was me and that one day it would all magically return, or so I hoped.

Now today, reflecting on the past few months, I can see that it did come back, and wow, is it back big time! I felt a new energy, a new masculine spirit around me, and that was when my daughter, Emily, suggested that I write this book.

Ever since, my life has now divinely fallen into place! By sharing my wisdom and connecting with the love of my family, I have healed, and I am experiencing the best years of my life so far.

Remember: you are never alone in this life. Just reach out and life will be there.

Have you ever felt an energy around you that you cannot explain?

Have you heard a voice in your head that wasn't yours?

Do you feel thoughts coming to you, but they haven't come from you?

Do you talk with a loved one who has passed that you were close to?

"To be yourself in a world that is constantly trying to make you something else is the greatest accomplishment."

Ralph Waldo Emerson

59

Be you-nique

Many of us don't see ourselves as unique, and that is probably in a large part down to how we were brought up. We were forever being told, "No, you can't do that." It is no wonder that we grew up trying to fit in because we weren't appreciated for who we were, the ideas we had, and we also never felt like we fitted in.

As adults, we compare ourselves to other people who are in the same profession, doing what we consider the most amazing things and not for a minute considering that we could be as good and as well-known as they are. So, we end up not living into who we really are but a lesser version of someone else who is usually famous.

At last count, there were over 8 billion people living here on earth. The remarkable thing is that no two people are the same. You might be saying, "That cannot be possible." But think about it.

They would need to have had the same two parents; the same family; the same circumstances; the same experiences as yours. Let me say it again: no two people are the same. Amazing – but true!

You are unique, and what you have to offer is unique to you. I believe that there are people waiting for, or even needing, your service. So, sit back and think about that for a moment and appreciate yourself for who you are, what you have learned, and the experiences you have had to bring you to who you are here, right now.

You can forever forget about comparing yourself to anyone who you see is providing the same thing as you. You bring your perspective with your learnings and experiences to what you want to do. No one else is doing the same thing as you nor even in the same way.

We live in a society that is bombarded with images of how we should dress and what we should look like, what we should be eating and the things we should be doing.

There is constant pressure to be someone who we are not. We are not encouraged to be ourselves and appreciate ourselves for who we are or what we want to be in the world.

So, maybe it is time to stop denying who you are and go forth. Be bold and use your uniqueness to do what you love, serving the people who are waiting for you.

Sit back for a moment and imagine who you want to be, without limits and other people's voices in your head. What do you look like? What are you doing? What are you feeling? Who are you serving? Welcome to your new life!

What makes you unique?

Who are the people you want to serve?

Do you appreciate your gifts and talents?

What do people say you do best?

"A compliment is verbal sunshine."

Atharva Veda

60

Compliment people

Most of us are uncomfortable receiving compliments and love from others. The unfortunate truth here is that by doing this, we are denying the pleasure, intention, and love that someone else is offering us. At the same time, we keep ourselves small and undeserving when we don't accept the compliment given to us. Most of us, more than likely, will give a compliment back rather than gracefully accepting that which is extended to ourselves.

Giving compliments to people demonstrates care and compassion for others. Genuine compliments require a shift in mindset to notice the good things that are happening around you.

As a society, we are conditioned to look for what is wrong rather than what is right. The fact is we do not have to be constantly on alert for danger as our ancestors needed to be, and so it requires that we have a mindset change so that we notice there are good things that are happening around us now.

As children, most of us were probably reprimanded for what we did wrong more often than we were admired or recognised for what we did right. So, it is no wonder that as adults we are wired to notice what others do wrong rather than notice the things that people do right, much less compliment them for it.

But it doesn't have to be that way. We can rewire our brain so that we notice the great things that are happening around us. The child saying thank you, the man allowing the woman to go through the door first, or the warm greeting from the checkout person and you spontaneously want to compliment them.

People underestimate the power a kind word can give to someone. Maybe the bus driver is having an off day, or a co-worker had an argument with their partner before they came to work. No matter what has happened, a compliment can turn their day around. Even the smallest compliment has the potential to change someone's day from disastrous to amazing and put a smile on their face. That is the power of a compliment!

Neuroscientists have found that the brain processes verbal affirmations the same way it does with financial rewards. The basic need to be seen, recognised, and appreciated by others is something we all desire. A compliment can lift someone's mood and impact their wellbeing, and at the same time, it has benefits for the person giving the compliment as well.

Giving compliments can also help build stronger relationships. Nobody likes being corrected all the time. By complimenting your partner, you are seeing the good in them so they will naturally want to do more.

Go on – try it for yourself!

When was the last time you gave a compliment to someone?

When did you last receive a compliment?

How did you feel?

Do you just stay in your own world oblivious to other people?

"My life is 50% wondering if it is too late to drink coffee and 50% wondering if it is too early to drink alcohol."

Unknown

67

Limit alcohol & coffee

I want to make it clear from the start that as I am talking about alcohol, I am not referring to just having one or two drinks occasionally. If you are otherwise healthy and drink moderately, it can, in fact, make you less likely to have a heart attack, stroke, or hardened arteries as small amounts can raise the good cholesterol levels.

Saying that, alcohol is a toxic and psychoactive substance on which you can become dependent, especially if you drink too much of it. For many people today, drinking is part of their daily routine, whether it's work drinks, celebrations, or get-togethers, not to mention when they get home from work and feel the need to relax. So, it is easy to overlook the health and social damage that can happen as a result since it has become so normalised.

The endocrine system is made up of glands that make hormones. They are the body's chemical messengers carrying information and instructions from one set of cells to another, influencing almost every cell, organ, and function of our bodies. Alcohol is one of the fastest ways to damage the hormone balance, raise oestrogen and cortisol levels while lowering testosterone.

Among other health problems, excessive drinking can lead to heart disease, stroke, liver disease, high blood pressure, and digestive problems. Anyone for a drink of water!

Those of you who are coffee drinkers will breathe a sigh of relief that coffee isn't as damaging as alcohol. However, after my experience with my sleep pattern when I had my café, I am not so sure that it can be exonerated completely.

The problem is drinking coffee first thing in the morning when your cortisol levels are naturally elevated. It is your natural fight or flight response to ward off any danger that may be there and can help regulate your blood pressure and blood sugar levels. Having coffee when you wake up can disrupt the natural flow of your cortisol.

Having an elevated level of cortisol for too long may suppress your immune system, making you more susceptible to colds and other contagious illnesses. It can also slow your digestion and sometimes not even allow the digestion of food, resulting in your body not receiving all the food's nutrients.

For some people, drinking many cups of coffee a day can cause insomnia, an increased heart rate, headaches, irritability, and muscle tremors. Like all things, coffee needs to be taken in moderation, so the balance of your body is not compromised in any way.

Do you feel a need to drink every night?

Can you stop at one or two drinks?

Do you need a coffee first thing in the morning before you can function for the day?

Do you drink coffee at night?

"We must use time as a tool,
not a couch."

John F Kennedy

62
Make the most of your years

Most of us would probably say that they think they have lots of time. "I don't need to do it today; it can be done tomorrow! or, "I don't need to call them today, it can wait," or, "I will fix that on the weekend" – all of which leads us to procrastinate because as we all know, tomorrow never comes.

It seems to compound as we age because time seems to speed up faster and faster until we realise it one day and wonder, 'What did I do with those 30 years?'

We become so caught up in our day-to-day life that the things that are truly meaningful to us keep getting put off, making it easy to lose sight not only of what has meaning for us but the bigger question of our purpose.

So, consider this my friends! If you are lucky enough to have another 40 years on this planet, then that equates to 14,600 days. Put like that, some of you are likely to think, "Wow, that's a lot of days."

You could look back on the past 20 years or 40 years and think about how fast they went. Think about how you use time now, and if you are wasting time, then maybe it isn't as much time as you first thought.

Of course, you can choose how you want to pass those days, but if you have goals and milestones to achieve, then you need to use your days wisely. Let's face it, it could end tomorrow for all you know. If that were the case, would you be content or would you be one of those who regretted not spending more time with your loved ones or didn't do enough of what you loved?

It is time to embrace the time you have left and be your extraordinary self and achieve amazing things. Take a reality check and find how and where you are spending your time.

Keep track of each 30 minute or 1 hour and categorise them according to whether they are (1) important and urgent, (2) important and not urgent, (3) urgent but not important or (4) neither urgent nor important.

You want to be spending more time working on things that are important and not urgent rather than tasks that are neither urgent nor important. The upshot is to make the most of each moment.

If you are retired, it needn't mean that you stop entirely. You can still be creative, have fun, do something meaningful, or even give back to the community in some way. I feel it is a great pity that so much knowledge and wisdom is lost because people retire and that's it! All their knowledge and wisdom isn't passed down to the next generation but goes with them when they die. Life is a gift and too good to be wasted!

Are you content with how you spend your time?

Do you know what you spend your time doing?

Are there times when you waste time?

Do you feel fulfilled at the end of each day?

"Water is life, and clean water means health."

Audrey Hepburn

63

Purify your H2O

We know how vital water is for our body since we are made up of around 60% water. Every cell, tissue, and system needs water to function properly. Water helps you think, focus, and concentrate better. The standard recommendation of water is generally eight glasses a day; however, that depends on many factors including how heavy you are, your age, and what exercise, if any, you do. Since not all water is equal, it can be challenging to decide which one is best.

Tap water is a type of water which generally has been purified using chlorine. If you want to remove the chlorine, then let it stand for 24 hours or boil it for 15 to 20 minutes. The water from your tap often carries harmful things like lead, bacteria, viruses, pesticides, and other physical and chemical substances, and since it is impossible to remove all contaminants, there are acceptable levels set down.

Spring water and mineral water are both sourced from underground and should be free from any treatment. The minerals contained in them will differ depending on the ground that surrounds the springs. Mineral water supplies the body with electrolytes needed for hydration.

Alkaline water may be the healthiest water with a pH level of 8 to 9.5, whereas regular water is neutral at 7. It may protect your body from free radicals which are often linked to inflammation in the body. Although distilled water is safe, the purification process does remove vitamins and minerals from the water.

For so many of us, it is so easy to buy a plastic bottle of water. Apart from the harmful effects on the environment, drinking water from plastic bottles is detrimental to your health. It is also not recommended that you store water in plastic bottles. Research has found additives such as BPA and phthalates can leach into drinks stored in these containers, especially when exposed to heat or used for a long period of time.

Water from plastic containers may be a potential risk of interfering with our immune systems and fertility, and it may even pose an increased cancer risk. It is advisable to drink your water from a copper or a glass container.

There are many purification systems on the market now if you want to have a ready supply of purified water on hand. It would be best to do some research on them to find one that suits your needs.

Do you drink your eight glasses every day?

A headache can mean that you are dehydrated.

Do you use plastic bottles?

Do you wait until you are thirsty and gulp the water?

"Love and generosity creates an exchange of positive energy and fuels further love and generosity."

Sharon Salzburg

64

Be generous with your love

There is something special that happens when you feel love for someone, not just a romantic partner, or a friend; it could be someone you just met but feel an instant connection to, sometimes feeling like you have known them forever and you just know that they are going to be a friend.

That happened to me when I met a beautiful young woman from Colombia. The instant we met, we knew that we would forever be best friends. She has come to be like a daughter to me and loves me as much as I love her. We have fun together, share deep conversations that are inspiring for us both, and I get to learn from her as much as she learns from me.

It feels like you can achieve anything and that there is not a thing wrong in your world. It is the most uplifting feeling I can think of that I have experienced. You go through the rest of your day as if you have wings.

Generosity in love is not about keeping a scorecard or expecting something in return or denying yourself or self-sacrificing, but rather it is about being generous with your love for your partner or friends.

When we think about generosity, we think about giving gifts or our time to friends or family, whereas it is just as much about how we relate to the people we love, to ourselves, and to the world. It is about being willing to open up, to share our love and what we have with others and feeling the connectedness.

When we make the effort to be loving, it is an emotional generosity that we are giving, which is no doubt the main ingredient to any long-lasting relationship.

Nothing demonstrates our love more openly than generosity, but it needs to be done in the right way. If we give our generosity out of guilt or obligation, then we surely aren't giving it out of love. While love is generous, generosity can only be expressed through love, and we cannot love by keeping it all to ourselves. It compels us to share what we have with other people.

We can be generous with our love for someone by providing emotional support when they need it or cooking them dinner if they have had a stressful day at work or surprising them with a gift to show them you care. Sometimes though, we need to give love generously to ourselves by having a rest day, a massage, taking ourselves out to lunch, or just asking for help.

We all have an infinite amount of love inside us and when we are open to sharing it, not just with our friends and our families, but with the world then our lives will be changed forever.

What is your love language?

Do you know your partner's love language?

How do you like being shown that you are loved?

When is the last time you showed love to yourself?

"*If you ate today,
thank a farmer.*"

Unknown

65

Be grateful for your food

Unfortunately, we are so out of touch with where our food comes from that young children don't know that potatoes are grown underground, tomatoes grow on a bush, or even that milk comes from cows.

Many adults would be unaware of whether the food they eat is genetically modified or not or even if it matters and probably don't know that some fresh foods are sprayed before being imported into Australia to prevent pests and diseases from being introduced. If they are not deemed safe when they arrive then they are fumigated.

Because the food just didn't magically appear on our plates by being grateful, we are giving thanks and appreciation to all the people who played a part in bringing the delicious nourishment to our plates: this includes the farmers, the truck drivers, the people in the supermarket and – oh, we cannot forget the cook!

Saying grace before eating your food has a long history. It isn't hard to see why being grateful for food would have become a ritual our ancestors had. Sometimes there probably wouldn't have been much food, if any, for them to eat, so being grateful for the food that was there would have come naturally. It goes beyond religious and even cultural boundaries, and it doesn't matter whether you are giving thanks to God, a deity, or to the people who had a part in the food getting to your plate.

It is believed that there are physiological benefits to saying grace before our meals. People tend to eat more slowly, chewing their food more slowly which aids digestion, meaning the food is broken down completely in your stomach and you receive the full nourishment of the food you have eaten. When you don't chew your food well, then your body doesn't receive all the nourishment that the food has because some of it may go through digestion not fully broken down.

When you say grace before a meal, you are also more likely to recognise when you have eaten enough and feel satiated for longer when you eat your food mindfully. You may even enjoy better sleep, lower stress, enhanced overall wellbeing, and improved heart health.

Saying grace as a group allows us to have a stronger bond with each other and greater satisfaction with our life. Even if you are alone, you can still give thanks for your food. I believe, though, it goes beyond the food on our plates and connects us to all the people who played a part in bringing the food to our homes.

After all, food is how we fuel our bodies to be able to do all we want to with as much energy and enthusiasm as is possible. Being able to do that means it is important that I know where my food comes from.

Can you imagine having to walk kilometres to find your food?

Do you ever think about where your food comes from?

Do you take the time to be grateful for your food?

Do you feel grateful for having a stove and a refrigerator?

"If you had weak eyes, they needed exercise to get strong. Glasses were like crutches. They prevented people with feeble eyes from seeing the world on their own."

Jeannette Walls

66

Do your eye exercises

From around the age of 40, people find that their eyes aren't as strong as they used to be. Many of these eye problems are associated with working at your computer and having difficulty seeing text at close distances.

Looking at a computer screen too long can lead to eyestrain, blurry vision, trouble focusing at a distance, dry eyes, as well as headaches, on top of the usual neck and shoulder pain.

The best position is to be looking at the screen with your eyes about 5cm to 10 cm from the top of the screen because your eyes see more below than above eye level. Try to provide shade for windows so there is no glare.

I learned over 20 years ago that eye exercises are one of the best things I can do for my eyes. Our eyes are a muscle, and so they weaken if not exercised. Mine are stronger because of the exercises. If I don't do them for a week, I notice my eyes start to weaken.

The exercises strengthen your eye muscles by helping you focus, stimulating the vision centre in your brain so your eyes become stronger.

Every day, I roll my eyes in a circle as far out as I can, first in one direction then in reverse. Next, I move my eyes diagonally as in an X; I do this on both sides. Finally, I move my eyes horizontally from side to side and then vertically top to bottom. I do each exercise 20 times which takes about two or three minutes.

To check your progress, choose a piece of text that you have trouble reading before you begin exercising and then look at the same piece of text a week later. For me, it was a week before I could read the text clearly.

When you are working in front of a screen, stop every 20 minutes and focus on something that is around 6 metres away for 20 seconds. Gently cup your hands over your closed eyes without putting any pressure on your eyes until all the afterimages turn black.

If you know me, then you will be expecting me to mention food – and I don't want to disappoint you! Of course, good eye health is determined in part by the food you eat. Foods full of nutrients like omega 3 fatty acids, zinc, vitamins C and E, and lutein found in things such as salmon, green leafy vegetables, eggs, and legumes are great for the health of your eyes.

How long each day are you working at your computer?

Have you noticed your eyes are tired at the end of the day?

Do you stop regularly if you are working long hours at your computer?

Are you nearing the age of 42 years and 10 months?

"I have learned that there is more power in a good strong hug than in a thousand meaningful words."

Ann Hood

67

Hugs, hugs, and more hugs

Now more than ever people are living disconnected lives. So many of us are isolated, living away from family and friends, and yet the world around us is busier than ever; people are stressed and lacking the social and especially physical connection that having a close circle of friends provides. While people are connected through social media, it doesn't give the one-on-one contact that we need to thrive.

There are two systems of touch. One is "fast touch," a system that quickly allows us to detect contact, like when we have touched something hot. The other one is "slow touch," which is a system of nerves called C-tactile afferents that process the emotional meaning of touch. They are seen as the neural input stage, signalling the positive aspects of interactions like hugging.

Hugs are such a powerful way to tell us we are loved and cared for, without the need for words. When we are feeling down, a hug can make us feel like everything will be OK. A hug from a loved one can ground us, reduce cortisol – the stress hormone – which is responsible for so many issues like obesity, low immunity, and sleep problems among other health issues. The effect of hugging has been found to lower our heart rate, reduce inflammation, and improve the healing of wounds while boosting self-esteem and making us feel safe.

Hugs increase certain hormones in our body and brain. Dopamine is the feel-good hormone that lifts our mood, controls anxiety, and fights disease. Oxytocin helps us feel calm, boosts heart health, and lowers our blood pressure, and through hugs, we get boosts of oxytocin helping us heal feelings of loneliness and anger.

Our immune system is strengthened by having hugs through the pressure on our sternum and, together with the emotional charge we get, it stimulates the thymus gland which regulates the production of white blood cells keeping us healthy. The therapist Virginia Satir said that we need four hugs a day for survival, eight a day for maintenance, and twelve hugs a day for growth.

It is interesting that touch is the first sense to activate in the womb at around 14 weeks. From the moment we are born, the loving caress of a mother and father has many health benefits including lowering the baby's heart rate and promoting brain cell connections.

So, who is up for a hug?

Have you had a hug today?

Do you do a quick hug and pat on the back or are your hugs longer and deeper?

Are you present when you give someone a hug?

How do you feel after someone has given you a long hug?

"If you listen to your body when it whispers, you won't have to listen when it screams."

Rivercity Pilates

68

Listen to your body

Our bodies are incredibly intelligent. If you are in tune with it and listen to what it is telling you, then your life will flow more smoothly, and you will be healthier. Everything that happens in your body is feedback to let you know that you need to do something or not do something. Unfortunately, we are not taught this, so people who don't recognise the symptoms will inevitably suffer later.

We are so adept at putting up with niggling pain, the tension, or saying "yes" to the boss, even though you are exhausted. We've been encouraged and programmed to just get on with our lives without looking at what our pain or exhaustion is telling us. This awareness is so important if we really want to improve our health and understand our bodies more.

A couple of years ago, I was madly trying to fit in so much it was more than I could handle. I had said to some friends who were working late that I would bring dinner over to them. If I had listened to my intuition, I would have cancelled it, but I didn't, even though my friends would have understood if I had.

As I was putting the food into my car, I slipped on a wet leaf (of all things!) and badly sprained my ankle. I still didn't cancel. I drove 25 minutes with the food, and by the time I got there, my foot resembled a football more than a foot. Of course, I was forced to have complete rest for well over a week. But the fact is I could have avoided all of that if I had only listened to my intuition and rested.

So, take a moment and check in on how you are feeling right now. Is there any tightness, pain, achiness? How are your energy levels? How did you sleep? If you are tired, then your body is telling you to rest because your nervous system is overburdened and needs time to recover.

We have an inner 'pharmacist' in our body which tells us what we need to do to help heal our body, we just need to tune in more often so that we recognise and do what our body is intuitively telling us to do. When you begin to listen to your body, you will start to notice things you completely missed in the past.

Do whatever you need to do, whether it is a gentle walk in the park, a heat pack for the pain, sitting on the beach in the sun, or taking a power nap. Of course, look at your diet: is it balanced? Does it support your body?

When you find the time to listen to your body, I am certain that you will be surprised by how much your body will tell you.

If you are tired, do you push through it and continue?

Have you unconsciously heard your body tell you something and you ignore it?

Do you continue eating even after you know you are full?

If your eyes are tired, do you continue working on your computer?

"*Don't take life too seriously. You'll never get out alive.*"

Elbert Hubbard

69
Don't take life seriously

*D*o you rarely find time to unwind? Are you worrying about the small things? Do you find it hard to see the funny side? Maybe you feel like you are in a competition with others or time? Are these concerns interfering with your life or your relationships? If so, then consider that you might be taking life a little too seriously.

When you take life too seriously, you don't necessarily have a clear perception of what is possible. You may develop an unclear and hazy view of what is worth your time and energy because you have a narrow focus and do not allow for anything outside of that to be thought about.

When you are so busy being serious, you can easily miss out on the fun and joyful things happening in your life. If this is you, then please don't wait until your deathbed to see that you missed out on these moments. Focus on the unexpected benefits that can come out of you being late and having your son or daughter give you the best and longest hug ever. Think about the problem or the moment when something didn't go the way you wanted it to and consider this, will it matter in two years' or five years' time?

When you are too serious and stressed, it is easy to fall into the trap of comparing yourself to someone else who you may look up to or admire. However, that can set you up for feelings of unworthiness, stealing the joy and fun you could have in your life. If you are a person who sees the things that are wrong first, try looking at them in a positive way before you start searching for the negatives.

We're so often busy being busy that it's hard to find a time to pause to laugh or enjoy the moment. With all you have to do each day, you may wonder, "What is there to laugh about?" Yet laughter has numerous health benefits from reducing stress to boosting your spirit and improving how you relate and connect to others.

Setbacks will happen, but trying to be perfect can make the setbacks seem more overwhelming. Embracing your perfectly imperfect human self can help release a lot of pressure of living up to unreachable expectations. It's OK to make mistakes. Making them doesn't mean you're not enough.

You may be one of those people who have to plan every little detail, but sometimes the unexpected can happen, and that makes it even better – you just need to allow for that to happen.

How is seriousness showing up in your life right now?

Do you have any time in the day to be able to sit and be?

How do your shoulders, neck, and back feel?

When was the last time you had a massage?

"A thriving household depends on the use of seasonal produce and the application of common sense."

Olivier de Serres

70

Eat seasonally

H ow and what we eat has changed radically in recent times. We go to supermarket and make our choices from the vast array of foodstuffs that are on the shelves. But it hasn't always been like that.

Man had to go foraging in the bush for his food every day, before our modern-day conveniences like fridges were available. The variety of their food was dependent on what was growing at the time they were out searching and each season, the food changed as different fruits and vegetables would grow.

Now, we are confronted with a different scenario: the same foodstuffs on the supermarket shelves week in, week out. We don't have to wait for the season's fruits to arrive; they are there for us whenever we feel like eating them. Fruits are picked and put in cold storage for months before they even make it to the supermarket.

It is interesting to note that in pre-industrial times, people seem to have been free of issues like colon cancer, colitis, and Crohn's disease, which are all related to digestion. This is possibly in part because they ate what was in season during the year. One of the last hunter-gatherer people on earth has shown that our digestive microbes change with the seasons. In the Hadza tribe in Tanzania, researchers found that the gut microbes of the tribe members changed with each season – at the same time as the seasonal diets changed – and that some microbes almost disappeared from one season to the next.

The study carried out by Stanford University also found that the gut microbiome of the Hadza tribe is much more diverse than what is found in someone from the west. Microbes in the gut make enzymes that change from season to season to help digest the foods of each season.

With each shift in the seasons, soil microbiology changes, and the microbes on the roots, stems, and leaves of each plant also change with the seasons. When we eat the plants that grow in that season, we also take in the microbes that are on those plants, which help to digest the food.

Eating by the seasons provides us with the right foods to be digested by the microbes in the gut at that time. Food eaten in season contains the greatest nutritional content at its peak ripeness and is at its tastiest. Can you imagine being rugged up against the bitter cold of winter and eating an ice cream? Your body knows that it isn't the season for ice cream. Food eaten outside of the season can put your body out of balance.

Do you know what fruit and veggies grow in each season?

Do you have a local market where you can buy produce?

Do you notice that you prefer certain fruit and vegetables at different times of year?

Have you got space in your backyard to grow your own food?

"*Of course, I talk to myself!
Sometimes I need expert advice.*"

Unknown

71

Talk out loud

We all have our silent voice inside our head, giving us solutions, telling us no or yes to choices we want to make or just commenting on what we should or shouldn't do. There is no rule that says we shouldn't voice our thoughts. So why wouldn't we want to talk to ourselves out loud? It is perfectly normal. What are the benefits of it?

It is estimated that the average person has 60,000 thoughts per day. Broken down, that equates to 42 thoughts each minute! Now, I ask you, how many of those thoughts do you remember? What I have found is that talking out loud slows down my thoughts and allows me to review them. I have found that I am more likely to remember them too.

I feel that sometimes when I talk about an issue out loud, it gives me extra time to deliberate over it and offers me a different perspective. It makes me stop and feel into the problem in a different way from when I am just thinking about it. I guess it is the same as not struggling in silence. Talking about a problem out loud sometimes helps me work through the issue. In other words, it can be a great problem-solving tactic.

It is also a great way to give yourself a pep talk to boost your confidence if you need it or to motivate yourself to get something done. You can get a task done that you have been putting off. When you voice the task out loud, it makes it easier to focus and get the task done.

When you do speak out loud, you can use your name, giving yourself emotional distance to process the conversation more effectively. Oxytocin is released when you know you are being listened to, even if it is talking out loud to yourself.

Make sure that when you are voicing your thoughts you are doing it in a positive way rather than from a negative perspective, which isn't going to help you do a better job. Focus on your personal superpowers to build confidence and courage to get the task done.

Self-talk can help you make decisions more easily and motivate you to do things you may be putting off. Keeping a positive outlook and talking to yourself kindly can have great impacts on your overall mental health as well.

Try talking to yourself out loud and notice the difference.

You normally sing out loud, so why not speak out loud?

Do you talk to yourself to seek expert advice?

If someone in the supermarket looks strangely at you, just tell them you're not ready to answer yourself back yet!

"There is more to life than
increasing its speed."

Mahatma Gandhi

72

Balance your busyness

*I*n these modern times, most of us are leading busy lives, and one of the things we take little time for is reflection on how we are living our lives. Compared to centuries ago when we needed to constantly be on the alert to threats to our safety, today that is not necessary.

Back then, a small mistake or letting your guard down could have meant death. However, today no tiger is going to jump out at us. We don't have to always be aware of danger as our ancestors were.

So, one would think that our fight or flight response is not needed as it was for our ancestors. While it isn't needed now, that isn't how it is at all. We worry about bills, being late, problems at work, forgetting your friend's birthday, and all of these increase our heart rate, ready for the flight response. But where are you going to run to?

The reality is that being constantly busy doesn't allow us to see what is really in front of us. Maybe we're missing out on a beautiful woman wearing a gorgeous outfit that stops us in our tracks for a moment or a little child giving his mum or dad the biggest loving hug. We are missing out on the beauty of life. It is so easy to forget to appreciate what we have and the world around us when we are busy.

It doesn't allow us time for reflection of our life or ourselves. Reflection helps us to develop our skills by questioning not only what we do but how we do it. If a recipe didn't work for me the first time, I certainly wouldn't do it the exact same way the next time.

Reflection allows me to decide what to change so that the recipe is delicious as well as nutritious when I make it again. That applies to many things we do — maybe with a little thought and reflection, things could work out to be a better fit for you.

Just as importantly, being busy all the time makes it harder to find time not only for ourselves, but for other people. It is the connection we have with our friends and loved ones that makes life more enjoyable.

Be honest with yourself and look at ways to create a less busy life for yourself.

Maybe it means priortising the things you need to do that are important and delegating what isn't important. You could set aside time each day/week that you spend quality time with your children/hobby.

Do you have an imbalance in your work-play life?

What would you like to change?

When did you last have any me-time?

What would you plan to do?

"Proper storage of food prevents it from spoiling."

Unknown

73

Store your food safely

Food poisoning is frequently caused by bacteria from foods that have been incorrectly stored, prepared, handled, or cooked. If food is not stored properly, the bacteria in it can multiply to dangerous levels. The danger is that food contaminated with food poisoning bacteria may look, smell, and taste normal. If you take care when you buy, handle, and store food it can not only reduce the risk of food poisoning, but it will last longer.

Cooked rice is one of the most well-known foods that needs to be refrigerated as soon as possible, ideally within two hours after it has been cooked. Onions and garlic are best kept in the pantry because the dry air in the fridge will dry them out and affect their texture and flavour. If you want to keep onion that has been cut up, then make sure you seal it in a container before putting it in the fridge.

Store cooked food above uncooked food in the fridge and check the temperature of your fridge, especially in summer. Make sure that there is air space round the food for the cold air to circulate. It is best to store cooked food in glass containers rather than plastic. Refrain from putting opened cans of food in the fridge as the metal will start rusting quickly and then contaminate the food.

Tomatoes and avocados are best kept at room temperature, but if you want to keep them after they have been cut, then store them in the fridge. Before putting avocados in the fridge, you can sprinkle some lemon juice on the cut and store it in an airtight container.

Neither tomatoes nor avocados ripen when cold. Treat bananas the same. The cold can make them go mushy and soft. If the bananas are starting to go brown, you can peel them and put them in a storage container or maybe even freeze them for ice cream or smoothies.

People tend to put a lot of things in the fridge that don't need to be there. Sauces, pickles, relishes, and jams are full of preservatives that don't need to be refrigerated. A good rule of thumb is if they are low-salt or low-sugar products or contain fresh vegetables, dairy, or eggs, then they are best refrigerated. Otherwise, they can be kept in your pantry.

When you bring home any wheat, grain, or rice products, place them in the freezer for two or three hours. This will kill any pests that might be in the packets.

Do you chill food as soon as you have finished eating?

Have you checked the temperature of your fridge lately?

Do you keep check of when the food was cooked?

Do you store cooked food above the uncooked food
in the fridge?

"Never give up on a dream just because of the time it will take to accomplish it. The time will pass anyway."

Earl Nightingale

74

Celebrate your life

*O*ur journey through life isn't as one directional or linear as we would like to think! We don't get through life without twists and turns, bumps, and steep climbs. We are always going to have these learning curves and trying experiences. They are what helps us grow and shape us into the people we become – and our journeys are unique.

My journey to now is probably nothing like what you have experienced in your life. Every event we have been through and all that we have faced and felt has shaped our perspectives, our interests, what matters to us, and what drives us, and not a single moment of this is or has ever been out of order.

Like it probably was for many of you, the first ten years of my life developed many of the beliefs I now hold. Being part of a family of nine was a great experience in many ways, full of learnings about who I am, sharing life with other people, and discovering how to get along with and understand different people. As one can expect, in a large family, one doesn't necessarily get along with everyone else!

It was after my dad passed and I was in high school that I really began to feel lost. At the time, I felt like I was on the outside most of the time, not really fitting in anywhere. I was searching without knowing exactly what I was looking for.

High school was challenging since unknowingly I had put a wall up to keep my heart safe, especially after my first friend I made in the first few weeks died in a car crash. Because of that grief, I decided that making friends was difficult and that it wasn't safe to love openly. I am also sure that I gave my poor mum many sleepless nights over the things I did during my journey of becoming as I challenged almost everything.

The turning point for me came when I was 19 years old. I was feeling down and depressed, standing on the cliff top ready to jump. Then everything changed. As I stood there, I happened to look up into the cloudless starry night and saw the brightest star shining down on me. In that moment, I felt my dad's presence and knew in my heart that jumping wasn't an option. It was the first conscious spiritual realisation I had that my dad was always there with me, guiding me in my difficulties.

That twist in my journey became one of learning all I could to be the best version of me. Of course, it still wasn't a straightforward path, as there were so many lessons I had to learn yet, especially in relationships. That was never going to work, but I tried three times (three marriages!) before I realised that! Okay, so I was a slow learner!

The last twenty-five years I have spent studying different courses and teachings in self-development that has taken me to where I am and how I feel today: completely at one with who I am and what I am doing in the world.

My wish for you is to reach the point where you are comfortable in your own skin, knowing who you are and doing what you love. It is that you are getting the most out of your life, so that at the end you will be able to say that you have lived to the fullest, with no regrets. And it is that you will embrace with an open heart each and every moment of the extraordinary journey of your life on Earth.

4 things I have learned:

How important it is to be present to enjoy all that is out there to be experienced.

Trust that you are always on the right path even though at times it doesn't feel like it.

To make the most of every moment as time is a precious gift that needs to be valued.

To express how much those close to you mean to you.

"Live life so completely that when death comes to you like a thief in the night, there will be nothing left for him to steal."

Kahlil Gibran

75

Live until you die

A lot of people work all their life and then, when they retire, they don't know what to do because they haven't made any plans at all. They have worked for around 40 years in a job that, in a way, has defined who they are, and some people will feel a loss of self-worth, having for so long been known as an engineer or a coach or whatever career they had.

Retirement for many will mean major changes to the daily routine. You may be thinking about how good it will be not to have to get up early and go to work – how good it will be to just relax and do nothing. That is OK for a short time, but it doesn't work for the long-term. We humans need plans and milestones all our life. It is what motivates us to get out of bed each day.

It seems to me that it doesn't matter how big or small your plans are, it is still important to have them. If you want to plant an oak tree, then do it, even if you won't be around to see it mature. It is the pleasure you get from having planted it and the benefits to your wellbeing that makes it important that you did.

The problem is that time is a finite resource, and when you are working, it feels like it is in short supply; therefore, you tend to plan how to use it. However, when you retire, there is suddenly an abundance of time, so, people feel that there is no urgency to use it wisely.

People who do nothing are at risk of becoming bored and depressed, especially if they don't have a strong social network. Daily routine and activities add purpose to life.

If you are approaching retirement, then there are some things that you could do, giving you new opportunities for a rewarding and even exciting retirement. Being active and social is a great way to ensure your mental and physical health are maintained all throughout your retirement.

There are lots of ways to keep active: find a new hobby that's rewarding and enjoyable; volunteer at any one of your local organisations who are always looking for people to support your local community; apply for a part-time position, especially if you want to learn new skills. Any one of these options will allow you to make new friends and do wonders for your health overall.

You could start a new business – or even write a book!

Do you truly live each day fully?

Do you have plans for the next year?

Do you have any goals you want to achieve?

What would you like to change?

"Twenty years from now you will be more disappointed by the things you didn't do than by the ones you did. So, throw off the bowlines. Sail away from the safe harbour. Catch the trade winds in your sails. Explore. Dream. Discover."

Mark Twain

Conclusion

Wellness is a journey we can all take. Caring about your life and health is one of the most important things you can do for yourself. It is a journey of learning and growing. When you learn something new, you want to apply it. Try it, and if it works for you, adopt it, and grow in the process. If it doesn't work, you can adapt it, try it, and if it still doesn't work, discard it and try something else. You still grow.

I don't want you to think that I have perfected everything I do in my life to this point, for that is far from the truth. Like all of us, I am a work-in-progress. There are still areas of my life I would like to change or improve, like removing all the plastic from my kitchen, but in writing this book, I now appreciate how far I have come, as I would like you to do, now that you have come to the end of the book.

Take a moment to acknowledge yourself for how far you have come. List everything that you do and add another list of the things you would like to change. Remember, you don't have to take action on them all at the same time. They say it takes 21 days to form a habit, so try doing one a month and congratulate yourself for each one you take on. I promise you that your life, your body, and your relationships will be the better for it.

The truth is if you don't know yourself, then you cannot truly know what you want. Even if you think you know yourself, take yourself on a date and check in with the real you of this moment – see what comes up.

If you need to let go of your fears, then learn to express how you feel. Find the work-life balance that works for you, get to know yourself at a deeper level, and do not worry about what other people think, then do that.

My wish for you is that you take your life in your hands and, with your soul's guidance, mould it to how you would love it to be, knowing what the right path for you is, with no regrets. If you don't know what you would love to do, then that is another journey for you to take. Take your humour and inner child along for the ride and let your life be an adventure with no regrets at the end.

My love and gratitude go with you on your journey.

Please let me know how you go.

With love,

Mama Rae

About The Author

Hi, my name is Mama Rae, Universal Mum and Soul Food Chef Extraordinaire!

I believe in nourishing ourselves from the inside out: mind, body, and soul. I am a cook who prepares nutritious and delicious food with love. My mission is to teach people how to cook food free from gluten, dairy, and refined sugar.

I was fortunate enough to grow up on a farm where we grew a lot of our vegetables and had access to fruit from the orchards close by. So, the food was always fresh.

After I left home, I heard an interview with Vicki the Vego, during which she said, "Do you know that three days after a lemon is picked, there is no Vitamin C left in the lemon?" It was in that moment that I realised just how important eating fresh food was. I believe that cooking should be as easy as falling off a log and... FUN!

I am the mother of now-adult four children (and many adopted children from age 15 to 60!). I love all things spiritual and spend my time with people I love (often over a Mama Rae banquet) or in my garden with my veges and chickens.

I would love to connect with you!

You can find me on:

www.mamarae.com.au

Instagram: @mamaraessoulfood

Mama Rae's Soul Food (or Rae Antony) on Facebook

Resources

3

https://www.dailyom.com/journal/how-to-practice-gratitude-when-life-is-hard/?aff=910&ad=1&utm_source=google&utm_medium=ppc&

5

https://lifespa.com/body-type-quiz-dosha-ayurveda/

https://lifespa.com/quiz-whats-your-emotional-body-type/

8

https://www.betterhealth.vic.gov.au/health/healthyliving/water-a-vital-nutrient

10

https://www.healthline.com/nutrition/how-to-read-food-labels#misleading-claims

14

https://www.naturesway.com.au/articles/what-vitamins-should-i-be-taking

https://www.bbc.com/future/bespoke/follow-the-food/why-modern-food-lost-its-nutrients/#:~:text=On%20average%2C%20across%20the%2043,the%20nutrients%20

18

https://www.ewg.org/the-toxic-twelve-chemicals-and-contaminants-in-cosmetics

24

https://www.healthdirect.gov.au/sugar#:~:text=Consuming%20
too%20much%20added%20sugar,increased%20risk%20of%20
cardiovascular%20disease.

https://www.clinicskinhealth.com/skin-journal/signs-of-a-
sluggish-immune-system#:~:text=70%25%20of%20your%20
immune%20system,unbalanced%2C%20therefore%20
lowering%20your%20immunity.

30

https://www.betterhealth.vic.gov.au/health/healthyliving/
Chemicals-in-the-home

43

https://www.thewellnessway.com/
the-dangers-of-microwaves-and-healthier-alternatives/

55

https://www.scienceofpeople.com/friends-important/

57

https://www.seriouseats.com/
cooking-fats-101-whats-a-smoke-point-and-why-does-it-matter

62

Steven R Covey 7 Habits of Highly Effective People

66

https://www.ergolink.com.au/blog/how-high-should-my-
monitor-be-5-tips-for-the-right-monitor-height#:~:text=Both%20
positions%20can%20plac

www.ingramcontent.com/pod-product-compliance
Lightning Source LLC
Chambersburg PA
CBHW052009030426
42334CB00029BA/3149